SELF TREATMENTS
FOR BACK, NECK AND LIMBS

A new approach

by Brian Mulligan FNZSP (Hon), Dip MT

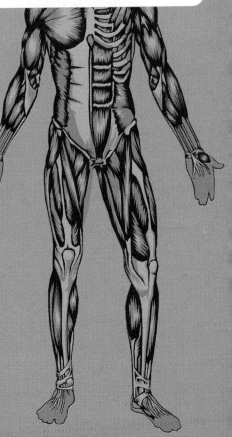

Published 2003

© Plane View Services Ltd, PO Box 14488, Wellington 6003, New Zealand

ISBN 0-473-09505-X

Printing and typesetting: Hutcheson Bowman & Stewart

The Author

Brian Mulligan qualified as a physiotherapist in 1954. He received his Diploma in Manipulative Therapy in 1972. He has been an International lecturer and speaker in the field on manual therapy for over three decades. Over the past 20 years he has developed his own concepts and treatments. His new approach has spread and is now being taught in most of the continents. Today he heads his Mulligan Concept Teachers Association. This international association was set up to accredit teachers of his concepts and to ensure that his concepts' courses were of the highest standard.

He has written and produced his own text-book 'Manual Therapy "NAGS", "SNAGS", "MWMS" etc.' and three teaching videos.

This book has been written to share with the public some of his innovative and certainly useful self-treatments plus some other management advice.

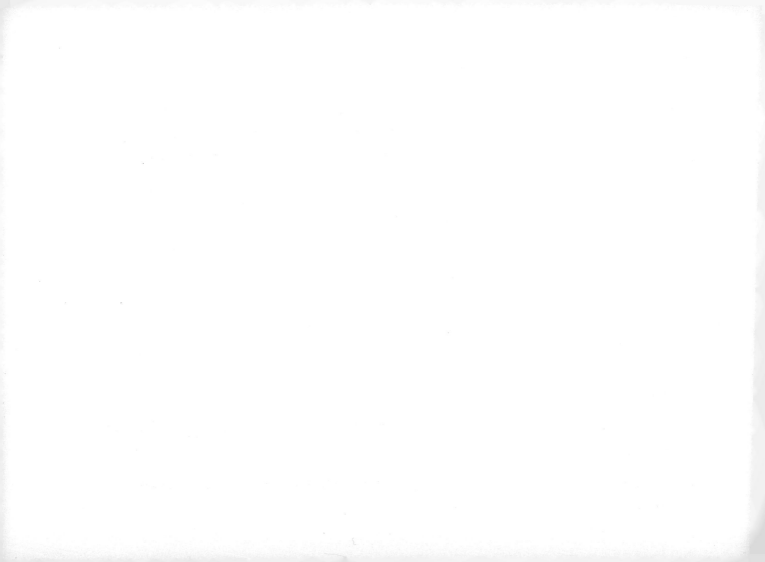

Acknowledgements

I would like to express my gratitude to Ron Stewart for reading this script and offering his advice as a lay-person. My wife Dawn and family have also helped with the text and photos. Thank you Denise Thomson of Hutcheson, Bowman and Stewart for your expertise. I acknowledge that the assistance I have received has been invaluable. Could I also thank colleagues and patients who encouraged me to write this text.

WARNING

There are many different causes of pain and not everyone responds in the same way to the various forms of treatment that are available.

If you suffer from very acute pain or chronic long-term pain you must seek professional advice from your medical practitioner.

Introduction

It has been suggested by many of my patients that I should write a small publication detailing treatment and management information we have found really helpful. Not to do so would be a shame because much of this information is not available to the public from other sources.

I have practiced Physiotherapy for over four decades but what makes this book pertinent is that over the last 15-20 years I have developed new treatment concepts and procedures. These have been professionally rewarding and exciting.
Self-treatments that have resulted from these concepts, form the bulk of the material in this book.

Many professions, like my own, osteopathy and chiropractic to mention but a few, have been mobilising and manipulating joints of the body for years. My main concept has been to combine mobilisations with active or passive movements. Apart from one exception, I have been unable to find in literature evidence of this approach being used by anyone else. The one exception was for the restoration of ankle flexion.

When treating the joints of the arm and leg, I call them *'Mobilisation with Movements'* abbreviated to *'MWMS'* and when dealing with spinal joints I call mobilisation with movements *'SNAGS'*. It is an acronym for 'sustained natural apophoseal glides'. The term *'SNAGS'* is less of a mouthful. The term *'SELF SNAGS'* is used when the patient is *'SNAGGING'* him/herself.

The two most satisfying things about this new *'Mobilisation with Movement'* concept are:

1. When it is used the patient will experience **no pain**. (Over 90% of my patients seek therapy because of pain.)

2. The patient should notice an immediate improvement in function.

Simply put if the technique causes any pain it should not be used. Try another approach. If there is no functional improvement at the time of delivery you do not proceed further.

Example. A middle-aged patient is unable to bend his knee fully because it is painful. A trial *'mobilisation with movement'* (*'MWM'*) is undertaken to establish if it enables him to bend his knee further and experience no pain when doing so. If it works then repetitions are done.

Another point is that most of this improvement should be maintained between treatment sessions, and where possible the patient is taught to do his/her own *'Mobilisations with Movement'*. Often the sustained mobilisation (or repositioning) can be maintained with a taping. As already mentioned this self-treatment approach using *'MWMS'* is the main reason for writing this small book.

Postural advice, tapings and other material will also be included in the text and at the end there are details of another new approach that I have developed called *'PRPS'* or *'Pain Release Phenomenon Techniques'*.

I have already stated that over 90% of my patients have come to me because of pain and they also have some movement dysfunction. Some examples of dysfunction would be that they may have restricted neck movement, be unable to flex up a hip sufficiently to climb stairs, unable to move an ankle freely after an ankle sprain or arising after sitting may be a problem. The list goes on and on.

Repetition can be tedious but please remember that with the exception of '*PRPs*', all the advice given in this book, when followed properly, should produce **no pain**. If the techniques produce any pain at all they would be not be used.

All the treatment and management advice, when followed, should not only produce no pain but when there is a loss of joint function this must also improve. If it doesn't there would be no point in continuing. There should also be a lasting effect. If not seek other advice.

If English is not your first language or if you have any problems understanding clearly the text then please seek professional advice.

Brian Mulligan FNZSP (Hon), Dip MT

Contents

Sleeping

THE LUMBAR SPINE

Many people with lower back complaints have problems in bed. When you have pain in bed at night the cause can be due to a chemical or mechanical process. I should explain that when we experience pain in our bodies the cause of that pain may be chemical or mechanical.

Chemical pain is felt when there is some inflammation irritating nerves and causing pain. Examples would be arthritis or appendicitis. Chemical pain can be treated with drugs, acupuncture, forms of heat or ice etc.

Mechanical pain is easier to understand. Examples would be a dislocated shoulder which has to be physically put back. A torn piece of gristle (meniscus) in the knee mechanically interfering with movement or a disc in the spine bulging and pressing on a nerve are two further examples. Mechanical pain can be dealt with, using surgery or some form of manual therapy e.g. manipulation.

When pain in bed is of mechanical origin there are several things that can be considered to see if they resolve the problem. The following suggestions *must* be beneficial. If they increase your pain or discomfort then do not use them.

1. The mattress. Is it firm enough? Lying on a sagging surface for any length of time can most certainly cause back pain. These days there are such a lot of excellent mattresses on the market and one should check these out. Some companies will often let you trial one of their products for a night or two. Take advantage of such a service and see if it makes a difference.

2. If you always sleep on the same side, as many of us do, try sleeping on the other side. Initially it may mean a few restless nights until you get used to it.

3. When you lie on your side, your waist tends to sag downwards because your hips and shoulders are much wider. Try sleeping with a small soft pad under your waist. This has proved useful with many patients. *See Fig 1.*

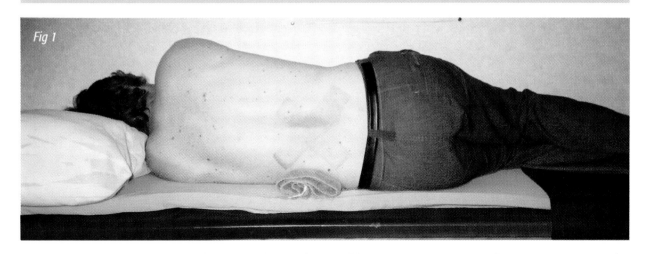

Fig 1

4. The safest way to sleep if you get night pain is to lie on your back with a very small pad under the curve in your lower back to maintain the curve. An alternative when lying on your back is to place two or three soft pillows under your knees. *See Fig 2 &3.*

5. If you get pain down the leg in bed, try lying on the good side with knees and hips at right angles. Now place at least two pillows under your feet to tilt your spine to the painful side. Try not to rotate (turn) your shoulders. If this pillow positioning increased the pain the technique is not for you. However it often takes many minutes lying in this way for the leg pain to subside. *See Fig 4.*

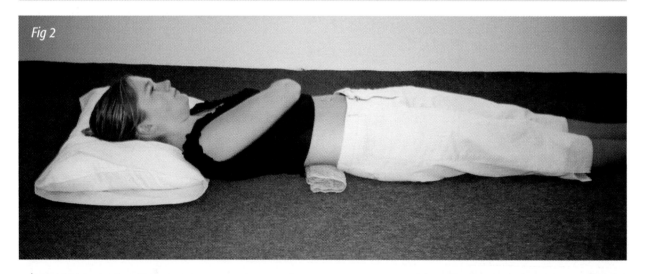

Fig 2

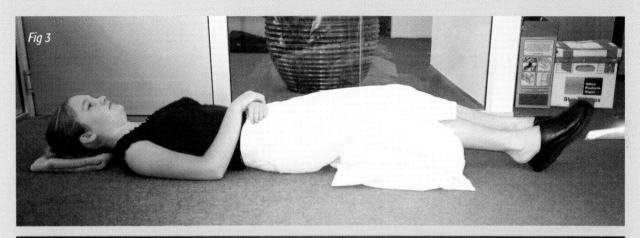

Fig 3

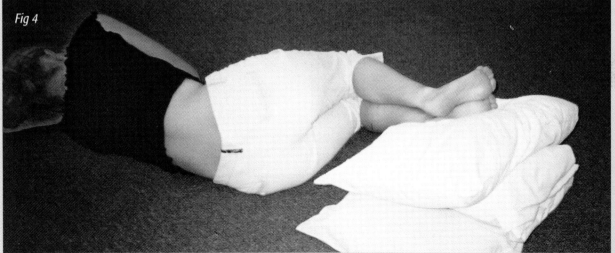

Fig 4

THE NECK

If you waken during the night because of neck pain or are stiff and sore in the neck when you arise in the morning, sleep in a 'pillow case' collar.

Take an empty pillow case and fold it in half lengthwise then fold again in three lengthwise. *See Fig 5.* It will now be about 6 centimetres wide. Wrap this around the neck so that it is at least double under the chin and fasten it with a safety pin. With this on, small ranges of movement are still possible in bed but the hurtful end ranges of motion are avoided. This type of support is not too bulky like a commercial neck brace and most of my patients have found it extremely helpful. *See Fig 6.*

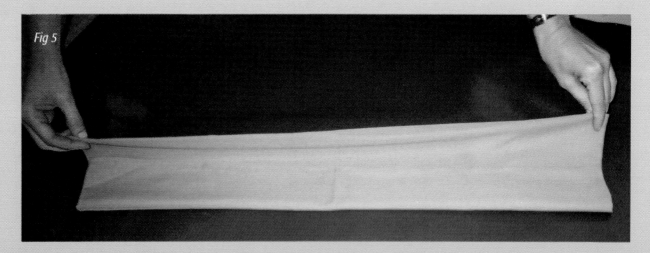

Fig 5

The pillow that you use is also important. It must not be too big or too small. You want your head and neck to be in line with the rest of your spine when in bed. If the pillow is too thick then your head will bend sideways towards your upper shoulder. If it is too thin the opposite will occur.

Pillows filled with feathers are wonderful as the content can be distributed to ensure you are comfortable.

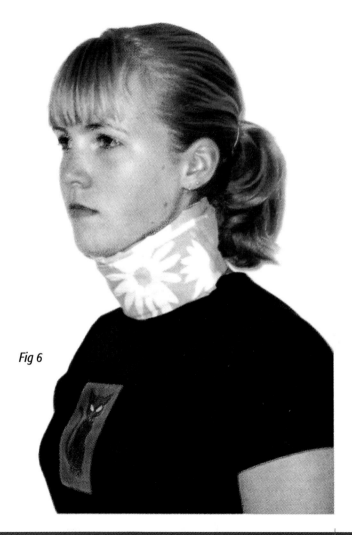

Fig 6

Sitting

Sitting is a big problem for those with spinal disorders. We are all encouraged to sit up straight and maintain the curve in the lower back (lumbar spine). When we do this our neck and head can be kept up straight and not jutting forward. Lumbar supports are built into many chairs, car and plane seats etc. Many types of portable lumbar supports are on the market.

The best advice that anyone could give of course, is never sit for too long. If your job involves sitting, get up frequently and stretch out. When watching TV every time the advertisements come on stand up and walk around the room.

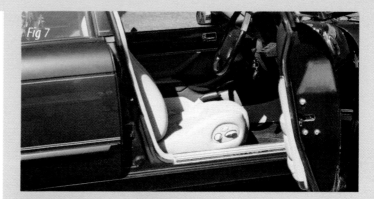

Fig 7

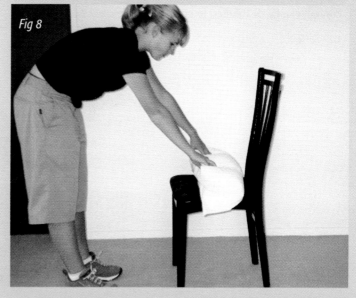

Fig 8

The added advice that I give my patients is 'ensure that the knees are lower than the hips when sitting'. Most cars for instance position the hips below the knees, which can make a lumbar support ineffective. It makes long car journeys an ordeal for back pain sufferers.

Inspect the lateral profile of your car's seat. *See Fig 7.* Sofas and easy chairs etc. are guilty of doing this.

The simplest way to get a better sitting posture is to fold a bed pillow in half lengthwise and place it on the back half of the chair's seat about 10cms from the very back. *See Fig 8*. Now sit on the chair ensuring that the sitting bones are comfortably settled on the folded pillow. Immediately, the hips are now higher than the knees and the posture is improved.

You should not feel that you are rolling forward on the pillow. *See Fig 9*.

A lumbar roll, if also needed, will now be more effective. Place a pillow thus folded on a dining chair at night and sit on this when watching TV. When seated properly the neck posture is also

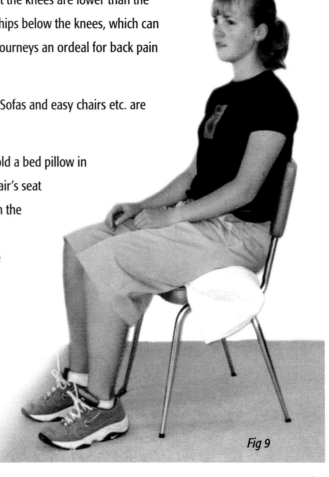

Fig 9

taken care of. If you sit before a computer, take a pillow to work and sit on it as described. The taller you are the greater the problem becomes when the height of the chair cannot be altered. For these individuals even with a folded pillow, the knees will be higher than the hips. A folded pillow may be too wide for an easy chair with the sides built in. Choose another chair.

When sitting, the folded pillow should be tried if you have a sore tail-bone (Coccyx). It is often called Coccydynia. This condition can persist for several weeks and sitting is always a problem. Most of my patients have found the use of a folded pillow on the chair as described above very satisfactory.

Another way of sitting with knees below the hips is to sit astride the chair with feet tucked back. *See Fig 10.* Not an elegant idea for the fashion conscious woman wearing a mini skirt.

There are of course chairs of the kneeler type. These are great for the back in that knees are below hips but can prove to be uncomfortable on the knees. The other point is that it is always nice to have something to lean back against and this is not the case with the kneeler chair.

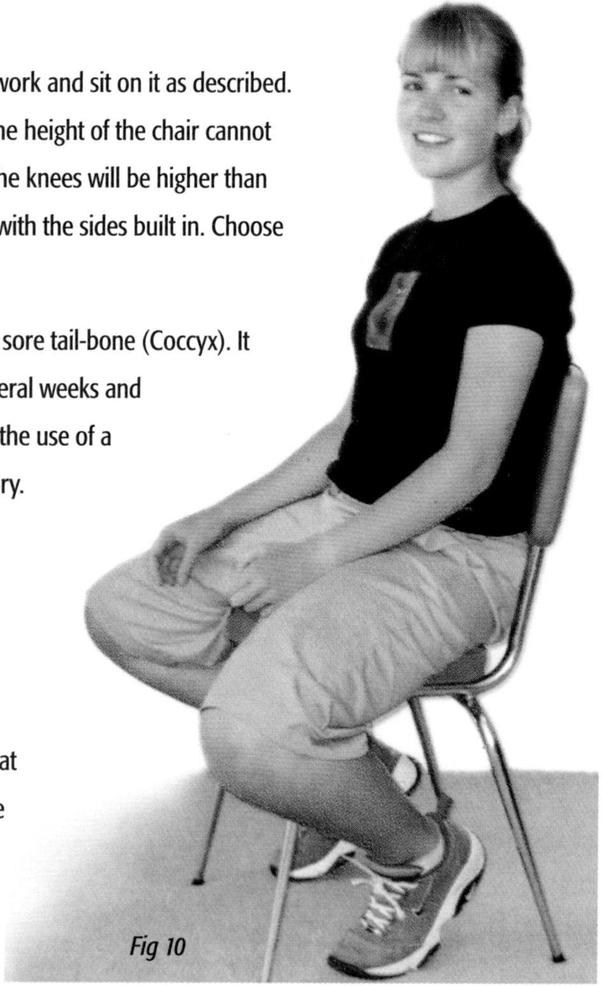

Fig 10

That computer screen really 'is a pain'. It draws our heads forward like a magnet and the end result, with regular computer usage, is upper back and neck pain and even headaches. *See Fig 11.* To stop this, I ask patients when sitting before a computer or TV screen to do the following…

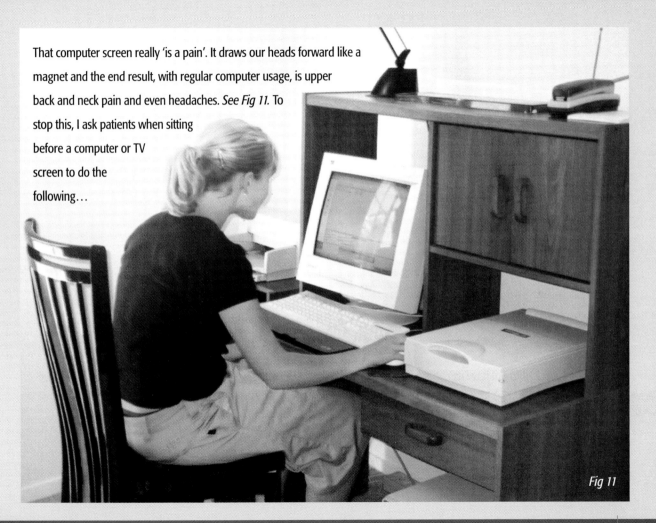

Fig 11

Firstly, sit on a pillow as already described and minimally tuck in or lower the chin. Now be aware of the distance from the chin to the front of neck and ensure that this distance does not change when staring at the screen. The head will not now be poking forward. This positioning is virtually impossible if the hips are below knees and you are unable to get a normal curve in your back.

On rare occasions you will meet patients who are pain free when 'sitting badly', so be it. If the advice given does not make an immediate change for the better, ignore it. Ensure of course, that the screen is in line with the eyes so they are not looking down or up to view it.

Most people working over a desk bend their lumbar spines, which can be a problem. *See Fig 12.*

I give further advice to the patient who is using a flat desk's surface for reading, studying or writing. In addition to using the folded pillow always flex over the desk by bending at the hips. For a change instead of sitting on the folded pillow when over a desk, come forward on the chair and flex your knees so the feet are under the chair. Now bend forward at the hips. *See Fig 13.* This keeps the back and neck straight.

If your lower back does not have its natural curve backwards it is virtually impossible to keep your head in a sensible posture.

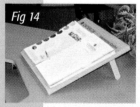
Fig 14

Ideal for those who are desk bound is to have an upward sloping surface to work on. *See Fig 14.*

Sometimes back pain with sitting comes from the Sacro-iliac joint. See the section on this joint. (*page 65*) If this is the case fold a small guest towel and place it under your buttock on the good side. When indicated your pain with sitting will stop as it reduces the sitting pressure on the side of pain.

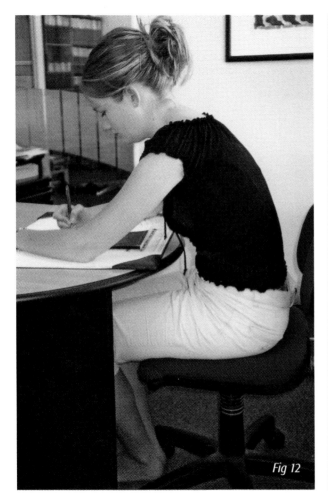

Fig 12

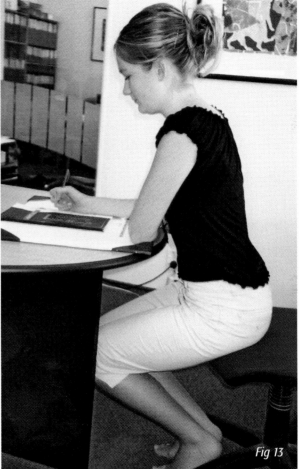

Fig 13

Exercises for the Neck & Shoulders

These days, exercise programs abound and there are many that meet the requirements needed to help those who are at a desk reading, writing or using a computer. My two favorites are:

HEAD RETRACTIONS

(taking your head backwards while the shoulders remain still).

This is done to keep the neck mobile and from becoming fixed in a jutting forward position.

Look at the side profile of older people. Many, with the passage of time, end up with their heads so far forward that they cannot stand up straight. With daily head retractions this horrible posture can usually be avoided. When done properly, the chin and forehead go straight back. *See Fig 15.* The chin does not move up and down at the same time.

The most important thing is that it **must not hurt**. If pain is experienced, ensure that you have a natural backward curve in your lower back and/or you can slightly alter the tilt of the head. Then take the chin back, or minimally rotate the head to one side, then retract. **These retractions should not hurt otherwise *do not do them*.**

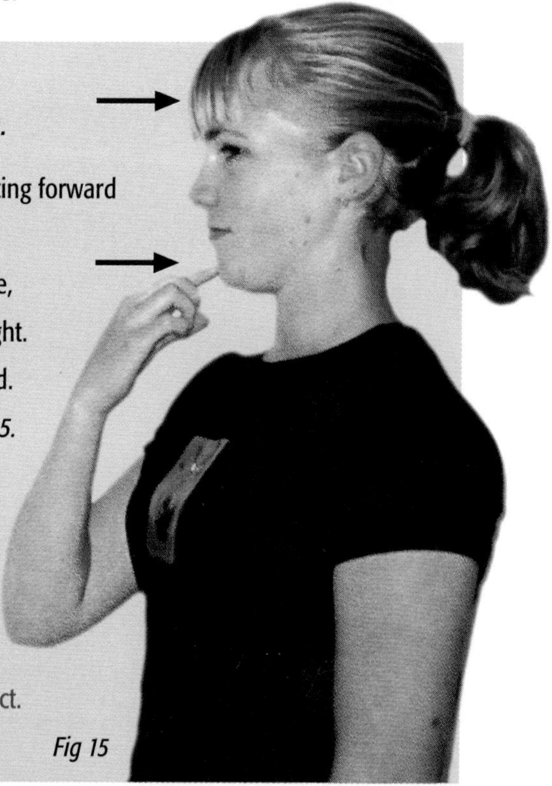

Fig 15

THE 'STICK UP' EXERCISES.

In movies and I guess sometimes in real life a robber may accost you and ask you to stick your hands up; that is why I use the term 'stick up'. With this exercise you may be standing or sitting. Take your arms backwards and then bend your elbows so that your fingers are pointing up to the sky. While maintaining a good head posture pull back your elbows and hands as strongly as you can. Keep pulling back and slowly reach up with your hands to the sky. *See Fig 16 and 17.* Pause for a moment and have a stretch up. Now while again pulling back your elbows and hands and keeping your fingers pointing up, slowly return your arms to the starting position. This exercise is repeated ten times at least once a day. It tones up the upper back muscles and stretches the tight chest structures. Very good for 'round shoulders'.

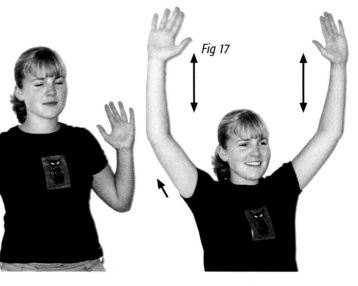

Fig 16

Fig 17

Sneezing

We all know of people who have 'put their backs out' sneezing. Many patients recovering from a l ow back problem can worsen their condition with a violent sneeze.

A good tip is to stand on one leg when you sneeze. Remember this in the hay fever season.

The Spine

I will deal with different sections of the spine, starting with neck – cervical spine (Cx), then lower back – lumbar spine (Lx), and finally the area between – thoracic spine (Tx).

See Fig 18

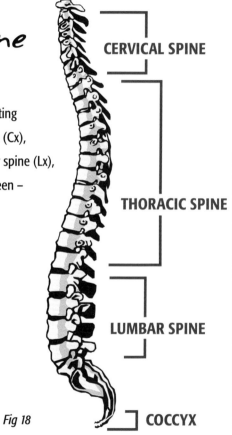

CERVICAL SPINE

THORACIC SPINE

LUMBAR SPINE

COCCYX

Fig 18

Cervical Spine (The neck)

HEADACHES

Millions of people throughout the world suffer from headaches.

There are many causes of these.

They can be due to serious pathologies but this is rare. However with severe, regular or continuous headaches one should always seek medical advice to rule these out. It is even more important that the doctor be consulted when children or the elderly have persistent headaches. X-rays rule out serious structural problems but other tests may be needed.

However, my experience shows that many headaches are from the top neck joints (upper cervical spine). When these are treated headaches disappear or are dramatically reduced in frequency and/or intensity. Hundreds of patients have benefited from my treatment and although I have a general practice, on one day a few years back I saw a record (for me) 22 patients who came to me with headaches.

Some headaches result from neck injuries like whiplash and others are posture related.

The offending posture is where the skull is jutting forward on the spine.

The joints that are most commonly involved are between the top two vertebrae. These are called the atlas and axis or cervical 1 and cervical 2. *See Fig 19*

These joints between the top two neck vertebrae are unique. All spinal joints below the top two, have discs between the vertebral bodies and behind these are two small joints, fingernail in size called facet joints. Between cervical 1 and 2 there are only the two facet joints. There is no disc.

All the vertebral joints below the top two have only very small ranges of movement, and rotation between them is restricted by a bony block. The joint between the top two bones is very mobile. There is no bony restriction to rotation. Ligaments, muscles and joint capsules limit the range of motion. In fact, when you turn your head to the right or left, half of the movement takes place between the first and second vertebrae. The rest of the movement is shared between the remaining neck and upper thoracic joints. When this top joint is 'sticky' or not moving properly, the

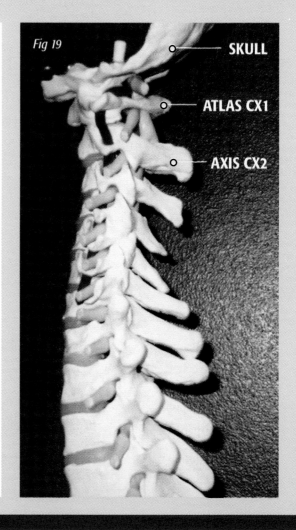

Fig 19

SKULL

ATLAS CX1

AXIS CX2

consequence can be headaches, sometimes giddiness and even nausea. This 'stickiness' is usually only detectable when the head is jutting forward and flexed. It could be from injury but is usually the result of prolonged periods of time with the head in a poor postural position, (sitting daily staring at a computer screen). When the skull slides forward on the vertebral column and stays there too long day after day it can cause problems. *See earlier Fig 11*

With headaches that are only one sided one would generally find a loss of rotation to one side only. With headaches that are felt on both sides you usually find the top joints restricted in both directions.

Movement restrictions, in these top joints, can be detected by a skilled therapist when the patient is lying or sitting.

When the therapist is testing NO pain, nausea or giddiness should be experienced. If any of these signs are present no further action should be taken. You should be sent to seek expert advice.

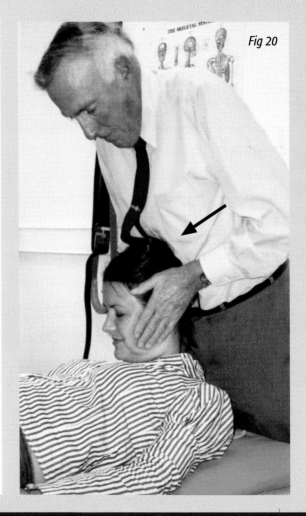

Fig 20

I will explain the way I test this area so that any skilled manual therapist reading the text would be able to do this.

To test this joint between the top two vertebrae, the patient must be lying on his/her back. The neck is fully flexed so the chin is on the chest and the head is rotated to right and left. When doing this the therapist keeps the head forward by using his/her abdomen. *See Fig 20.* I do not let the neck bend sideways or come out of this fully bent forward position while assessing it.

The other way is with the patient sitting. The neck is fully flexed and the patient pulls it further down with a free hand. Now they rotate to the right and left in this position. *See Fig 21.* This will show up a restriction when done properly.

Some headache sufferers have a loss of movement in both directions, others just in one. As already mentioned, when headaches are only felt on one side, the restriction is usually only to one side. When the joint range of motion is normal it will turn approximately 45 degrees in each direction. Some patients I have seen with nasty headaches often have as little as 2 or 3 degrees.

When restricted, there is a self-treatment technique that I will describe which should result in an instant increase in range of movement.

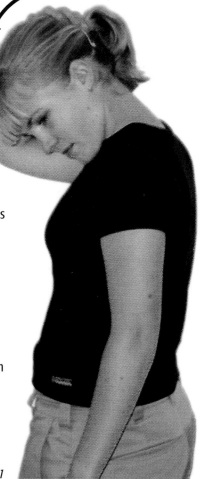

Fig 21

Before describing the technique, I must say that it would be wise to consult a therapist to assist you.

If you have a restricted joint then you could try this self-treatment called "SELF SNAGS".

Firstly if you are going to try "SELF SNAGS", there are golden rules that must not be broken.

"SELF SNAGS" **must not be used** when there is severe pain – nor on children, the elderly, the osteoporotic, the chronically ill, those with rheumatoid arthritis, those on steroids or after neck traumas that have not been checked out by X-Ray.

You **must not use** these techniques if you felt sick or giddy with neck movement or if your vision is affected in any way with movement.

The most important rule is that when applied there **must be no** pain, nausea, giddiness or visual disturbances. In fact you must be symptom free.

On the first day, the treatment technique is only repeated twice as a precautionary measure. If after this, all is well, up to six repetitions can be done on one, two or three times each day. Stop when symptom free.

On the following page is an illustration and text describing the self-treatment – "SELF SNAGS" – to restore movement to atlas/axis joint.

After "SELF SNAGS" the movement should be checked to ascertain that an improvement has been attained. If not then they are of no value.

SELF SNAGS

"SELF SNAGS" to restore rotation between Cervical 1 and 2 (atlas/axis) using a small towel.

The technique to be described is for a loss of rotation to the **right.**

When undertaken no nausea, giddiness or visual disturbance signs should occur or pain should be experienced. If there is any discomfort then the towel must be repositioned. It may not be high enough.

If not symptom free the technique must NOT be used.

Sit with a small towel around neck. Place selvedge (woven edge of cloth) (*See Fig 22a.*) on one side of the towel just below the base of skull so that it lays horizontal, just below left ear lobe and level with top teeth or just below the nose. Grasp selvedge on the end of right side of towel with left hand, and selvedge on the end of left side with right hand. (*See Fig 22b)* The right forearm should be on top of left. Hook bent left elbow on corner of chair.

The right hand pulls towel horizontally to move head round in right rotation. Keep head up straight and do not side bend. You should feel no pain if the technique is indicated and you are pulling on correct vertebra.

When you have pulled it around as far as it will go it is important to get your partner to apply firm but sensible overpressure to enhance the procedure. Never keep the neck in this rotated position. Return immediately to the starting position. An increase in range of movement should be the result when retested.

Remember NO pain!

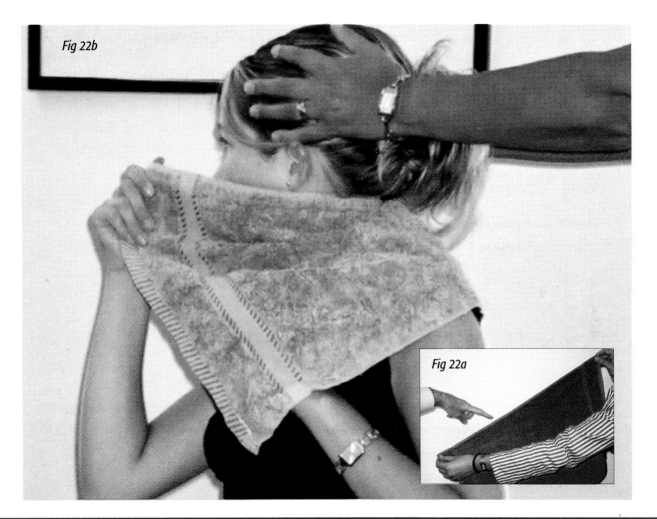

Fig 22b

Fig 22a

Repeat only two times on day one as a precaution. If OK on subsequent days repeat six times and repeat this sequence two or three times daily initially if necessary.

Stop when symptom free.

If range of movement is limited to **left** just undertake exercise with left arm on top and right elbow hooked on the back of the chair.

Neck pain and stiffness

I am now thinking of the patient who comes in with neck pain, which spreads across to the shoulders. It may be affecting just one side or both. They have movement losses and these movements are usually painful.

If this applies to you and provided you have no pain in arms, are sensible and remembering the concerns mentioned before with headaches the following procedures can be tried.

Remember none of these should cause any pain. If they do, STOP.

1. For pain with and loss of end range flexion (bending head forward).

I refer here to the patients who experiences pain and loss of the last few degrees of flexion. They cannot bring chin down to neck. If they have pain when initiating flexion they would not try this technique. This is for those with pain and stiffness towards the end of forward bending.

The technique is called **"fist traction"**.

If you are in this category, place clenched fist under your chin so that chin sits on the plateau formed by your curled index finger and thumb. Your curled little finger lies on upper end of your breastbone.

Now place your free hand on the top of your skull and pull head down and forward. *See Fig 23* .

Because bending of your neck into the sore range is blocked with your fist, painless traction will take place in the lower joints of your neck. You sustain this 'traction' for ten seconds and repeat three times.

After three fist tractions your neck should flex freely without pain.

This can be repeated six times a day if necessary.

Neck flexion can be quickly restored using this technique.

If after the first three tractions there is no change in the flexion range give the treatment away. Remember, no pain.

Fig 23

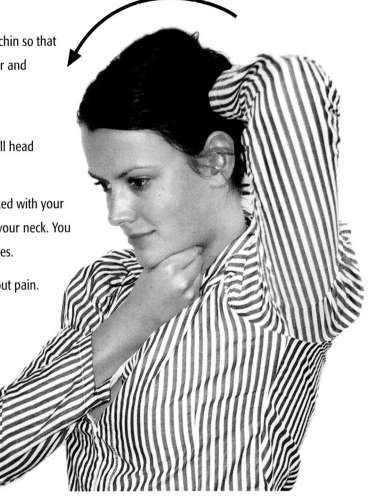

2. For loss of extension. (Tilting head backwards).

When there is very little extension one would suspect the upper joints in neck. When there is pain and a loss near end range then one would suspect trouble in lower part of neck.

The technique to be described is called a "SELF SNAGS" for extension. To do this you will again need a small towel.

Place the selvedge on one side of towel across the back of neck, just above the level that you suspect. Grasp end corners of the towel on same selvedge side. Now pull up on the ends of towel in direction of your eyeballs. Sustain this pull and slowly tilt your head back. As you bend your neck backwards your hands go with the head to maintain pull up in eyeball direction. *See Fig 24.*

If these "SELF SNAGS" are indicated your head will go straight back with no pain.

Do not let pull up with towel go until your head is again up straight. (Remember, when you try a "SELF SNAGS", no pain at all must be experienced. If there is any discomfort you may be at the wrong level and you could move the selvedge at the back of your neck up a centimeter or two.)

Do six times and then reassess neck to see if you can now bend back with no pain. If you can this is great, and the procedure can be repeated several times a day until you are back to normal.

This should only take a week or so.

Do not repeat the technique, if on first try, your neck pain and restriction is no better.

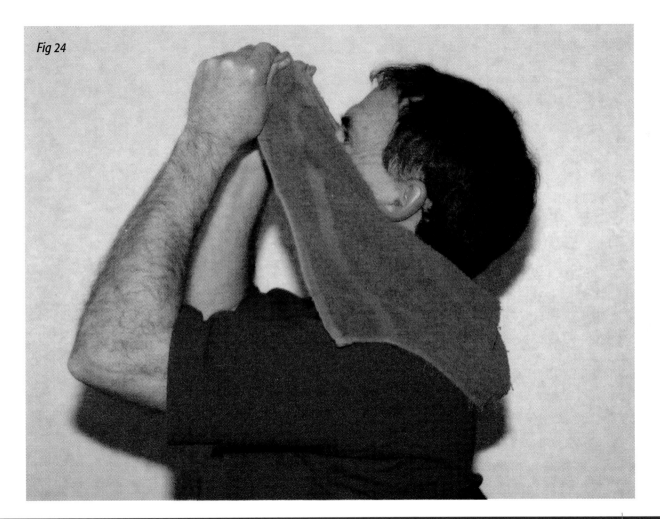

Fig 24

3. For a loss of head turning (rotation).

Those of you who have poor posture or sit badly at a desk or computer with your head jutting forward will eventually have neck problems. You will experience neck pain, which spreads across to your shoulders. It may be just on one side or both and with this discomfort there is usually some loss of rotation.

This technique is not for those with a gross loss of movement.

Provided pain is localised to areas just mentioned and is not severe, you can try rotation "SELF SNAGS".

The purpose here is to hook under a spinous process in the lower neck (where the stiffness originates) with the selvedge of a hand towel, lift it up to free the segment and pull head around with towel. *Figure 25/26.* Details follow.

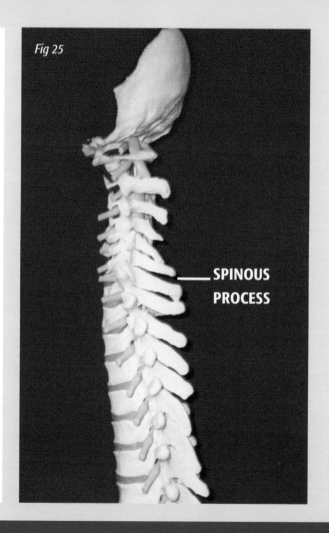

Fig 25

SPINOUS PROCESS

The technique to be described is for a loss of head turning to right. **Remember when undertaken no pain whatsoever should be experienced**.

If there is any discomfort then incorrect level may have been chosen in the neck and towel must be repositioned. If still sore then technique would NOT be used.

Sit with a small towel around the neck.

Place selvedge, on one side of towel, under the vertebra at the back, low down in your neck. Initially take it down as for as it will go.

Grasp end of the selvedge on right side of towel with left hand, and left side with right hand. The right forearm should be on top of left. Hook bent left elbow on the corner of chair.

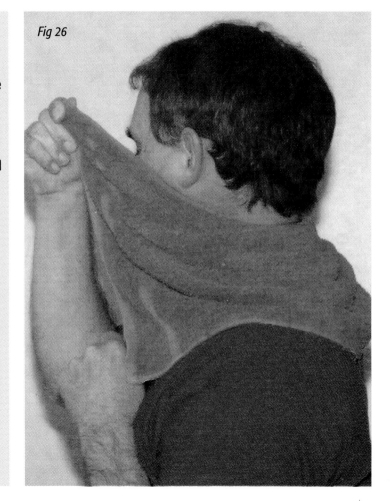

Fig 26

The right hand pulls the towel up in direction of left eyeball and at the same time pulls head round in right rotation.

It is important that head does not tilt sideways, forwards or backwards but remains erect. *See Fig 26* .

You should feel no pain if technique is indicated and you are pulling up on correct vertebra. If sore, shift edge of towel up about two centimetres. If still sore this technique is not for you.

It is very important (to enhance the procedure) that you get your partner to apply overpressure, when you have pulled it round as far as it will go. They must make it go a *little further* round but remember NO pain with this! (Never keep the neck in this rotated position. Return immediately to the starting position.)

After this self treatment the neck will have an increased range of rotation.

On the first day repeat twice only. After that repeat six times and this sequence can initially be repeated up to six times a day. It would be prudent to seek advice from your therapist regarding frequency.

If the range of movement is limited to left just undertake exercise with left arm on top and right elbow hooked on back of chair.

Sleeping.

Please do not sleep on your front (face down).

If you do, the chances are that you will eventually have neck problems. If you have a neck problem then sleeping face down (prone) can aggravate it. It is a hard habit to break.

My suggestion to patients who sleep prone or have problems with their neck in bed anyway is to sleep in a pillowcase collar.

I have earlier described how to fold a pillowcase to make a night collar. F*igures 5 and 6*

With a pillowcase collar on you will be unable to lie on your front because the neck cannot turn enough to allow you to breathe. With the collar on, extreme movements of the neck, that cause pain, are not attainable while sleeping soundly.

The Lumbar Spine (Lower back)

Today in the Western world you can expect to live for much longer than the biblical three score years and ten. During a lifetime it is highly likely that you will experience episodes of back pain. For some, these may be of nuisance value rather than disabling but some people have terrible episodes of back pain that may even require surgical intervention. When this is necessary it is nearly always the inter-vertebral disc that is damaged. You will note that I used the word episodes, as rarely would a person have ongoing pain, but once you have hurt your back the chances of it recurring are high.

There are many causes of back pain and even a greater number of different practitioners (orthodox and un-orthodox) claiming to be experts on the treatment of back pain.

Many 'experts' direct their therapy towards discs in the spine and others direct their attention to the little facet joints behind them. *See figure 27.* These facets are the structures that make an impressive click sound when manipulated. Manipulations have an important place and I personally have used them for many decades.

Patients are often told, when the sound is heard, that their spine has just been 'put back'. Few question this inaccurate statement and I cannot blame them even though that claim is nonsense.

After manipulation some do feel an immediate improvement while others are assured that any subsequent improvement will be because of the manipulation. That final statement would be hard to prove.

With recurring back pain, Australian physiotherapists have evidence that certain spinal muscles can be weak and need to be strengthened. Their research shows that when these muscles are strengthened your chances of a recurrence are reduced. Muscles with fancy names like the transverse abdominus and multifides are among the ones to seek strengthening advice for.

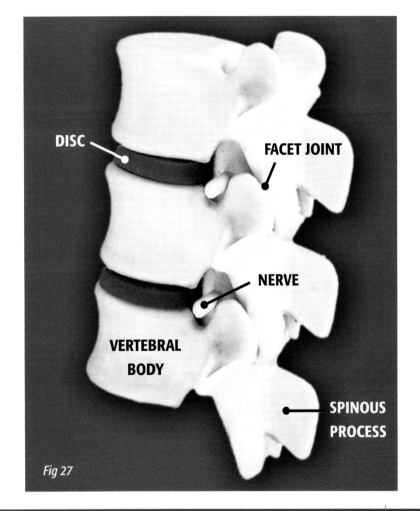

DISC

FACET JOINT

NERVE

VERTEBRAL BODY

SPINOUS PROCESS

Fig 27

Lifting.

When lifting, even with a normal back, there are three very important things you can do to protect your back. School children should be reminded over and over again to heed the advice below.

Firstly bend your knees.

Patients will say to me 'How can I bend my knees when picking up a wide clothesbasket or lifting a child out of a bath?' The message out there is that you must almost squat down. This is usually not possible but if you only bend your knees a few degrees it will still take a lot of the strain from your back when lifting.

The second bit of advice is to push your 'tummy' (abdomen) out sideways. When lifting push the muscles out sideways as you do when you grunt and keep them tight while you lift.

This helps to support your spine by giving you a corset of muscle. Nature is giving you a message when you have to grunt when you strain to lift something heavy. If you place your hands over muscles on each side of your abdomen just below your ribs and grunt you will feel the muscles tighten and shoot out sideways. Weightlifters do this. They often wear a belt around the waist when lifting. They push out sideways against the belt to protect their backs.

This action builds up intra abdominal pressure.

Using your muscles in this way, when getting in or out of a car or bed, or getting up or down from a chair, can make a tremendous difference when your back is sore.

Thirdly never lift a heavy or awkward object in haste. Take your time.

More specific advice on ways to lift objects is readily available from many sources.

LUMBAR STIFFNESS AND CENTRAL BACK PAIN WITH MOVEMENT

The assessment of a patient with a sore back is complex. It is difficult to suggest a self treatment for a patient that you have not seen.

There are risks with this approach so if you would like to try what I am about to detail, remember;

1. The procedure should not be painful. If there is any discomfort do not use it.

2. It must be seen to be beneficial. If for example you have a loss of backward bending, that movement should improve painlessly while you are using the technique.

3. If you have any health problems, you are 'getting on in years' or have any concerns please first consult with your medical advisor or therapist for advice.

4. When you first try a technique just do it three times on day one and leave it at that. Do no more to make sure you have no delayed undesirable reaction. The next day you can repeat the 'exercises' ten times, several times a day.

5. If pain that you are experiencing is severe and disabling seek medical attention and do not try these techniques.

6. If you have back pain and a lean to one side then you should see a therapist who is aware of the R A McKenzie treatment for a 'lateral shift'. There is no better approach for this condition.

Self treatment for stiffness and pain.

As we get older we can expect to experience some stiffness in our joints and that can be to our advantage. Our muscles do lose some of their tone and if our joints were too mobile we could have problems as a result.

The self-therapy that I am about to describe is called "SELF SNAGS". We used the same term when writing about neck treatments. "SNAGS" we said was an acronym which stands for 'Sustained Natural Apophyseal Glides'.

As a therapist I use "SNAGS" on the spines of many of my patients every day. They are extremely useful. When ever possible, we teach patients to "SELF SNAG" at home when they are shown to be effective.

With very painful backs, we delay the training of the patient until the pain is not severe.

For "SELF SNAGS" you will need a long belt like one of those we wrap around a large suitcase, or buy a 2 metre length of car seatbelt material.

1. Stiffness and pain with backward bending.

Let us assume that you have a central low pain in your back when you arch backwards.

Place a long belt across your back at lower waist level. It lies across what is called the lordosis. *See Fig 28a.*

That is the forward curve in the middle of our backs that is present when standing erect. It becomes humped when we bend over.

Holding each end of belt firmly, take your forearms forward, then bend elbows and take hands up to make contact with chest. The edge of the belt around your back should now be secured to the spine of the vertebra it lies over. Look at the illustrations. If the belt is long enough you can tie ends together so that you can grasp inside the loop and when you bend up your elbows the belt will securely pull up on chosen spinal segment.

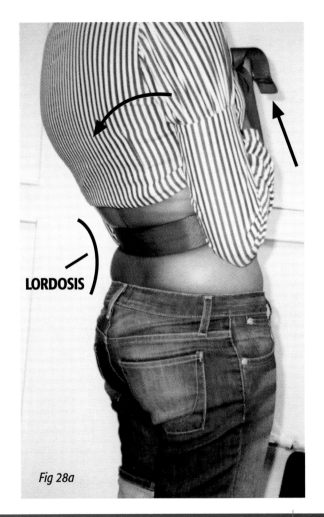

LORDOSIS

Fig 28a

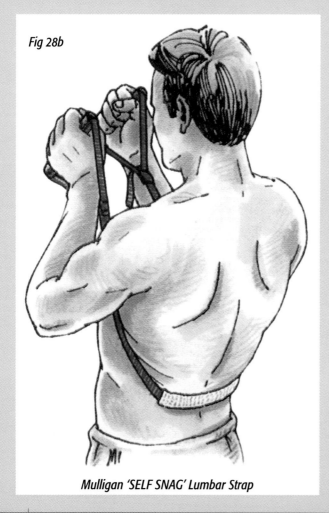

Fig 28b

Mulligan 'SELF SNAG' Lumbar Strap

The purpose of pulling up on belt is to unload or free the facet joints at that level and enable you to arch back further with no pain. Try this and see if your pain with extension has gone and you can extend further.

Keep your hands in contact with chest all the time.

If there is pain or discomfort you may be at the wrong level. Try again with belt about 2 centimetres higher or perhaps 2 centimetres lower.

If still sore, do not proceed.

As mentioned earlier, on the first day it is prudent to repeat the painless "SELF SNAGS" only three or four times as a trial to ensure there is no later discomfort from the exercise.

On day two if not sore repeat "SELF SNAGS" ten times.

Usually up to ten of these exercises with the belt can be repeated up to ten times a day as a treatment routine until you feel much better.

Sometimes with "SELF SNAGS", if the joint is really 'stuck', you will have no success with extending <u>backwards</u>. If this is so, bend your knees about 10 degrees, pull up on the belt as before, and bend <u>forward</u> provided there is no discomfort. This, in effect, will often free the segment so that you can now bend <u>backwards</u> further and without pain.

On the first day repeat three or four times only. After that you would repeat "SELF SNAGS" up to 10 times.

Remember that after these repetitions your range of free movement should have increased.

This approach with a belt or towel can be so effective that in the USA a firm called OPTP in Minneapolis sell a special belt with hand-grips that make the self-therapy much easier. *See Fig 28b.*

See my web page www.bmulligan.com **for more details**.

There is another way of applying "SELF SNAGS" using your hands and it is particularly useful for one sided low back pain with movement. You need a reasonable amount of strength in your forearms.

Firstly clench your hand (make a fist) on the side of your pain. You place the shaft of the bone from the knuckle and the first joint of your index finger to the side of your spine just above the level of your pain. *See Fig 29a and 29b*

Place your other hand under the one on your back.

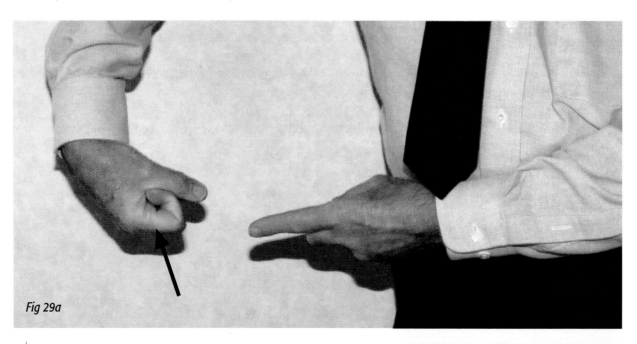

Fig 29a

The procedure is to lift up the spine on one side with the hands and maintain this lift as you arch backwards.

When indicated you will be able to move with no pain as is the case with the belt. I find that younger people cope with this technique much better. Remember if it is sore you try moving your hands up a centimetre or so in case you are on the incorrect level.

You can also use your hands in this way in the centre of your lumbar spine.

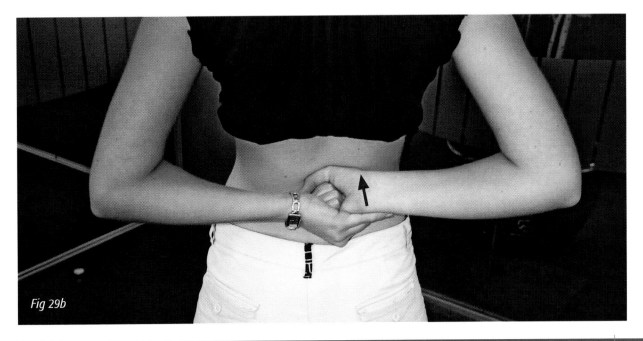

Fig 29b

2. Stiffness and pain with forward bending.

Provided the pain with bending is confined to the back and does not radiate down leg, you can "SELF SNAG" the spine as you did for backward bending. With your knees bent about 10 degrees you pull up on the belt and, if pain free, bend over as far as you can and then come up straight without letting go of the upward lift with the belt. *See Fig 30*

Initially just try three "SELF SNAGS" as a precaution to ensure all is well. Subsequently, sets of ten, several times a day, can be done. Intersperse with forward flexion "SNAGS", a backward "SELF SNAGS" to 'balance' the routine.

As with forward bending you can use your hands as described for backward bending.

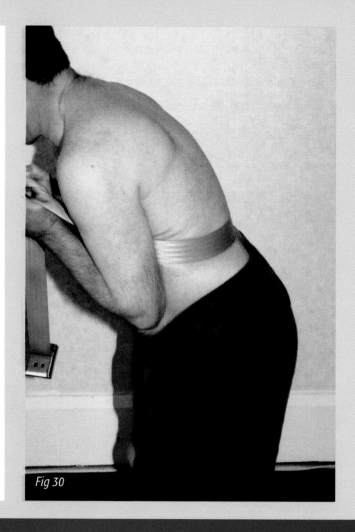

Fig 30

3. Stiffness and pain with side bending (leaning sideways).

"SELF SNAGS" with a belt can be tried, but because of the soft tissues that gather when we bend sideways, the treatment may not be successful. Using your hands on the restricted side may be better. However after repeated forward and backward bending, side bending is often much better.

The thinner you are the better because the belt can readily make contact with your bony spine. Those of you who are of generous proportions will not find "SELF SNAGS" as easy unless you can use your hands. You should see a therapist who is familiar with "SNAGS" and they would treat you. Size does not prevent the therapist from successfully "SNAGGING" you.

Don't you think "SNAGGING" is a lovely word?

4. A loss of 'straight leg raise' (SLR). (A technical test which is explained below).

A patient with a serious low lumbar disc problem will have a marked loss of 'straight leg raise' and pain produced with the test can be experienced down the leg as far as the foot.

Whenever the lumbar spine is examined by a doctor or spinal therapist one regular test is always done. It is called 'straight leg raise' (SLR). The patient is on his /her back and the doctor raises first one leg and then the other with the knee straight.

This is to see if the range of 'straight leg raise' is limited and if it produces any pain.

The range is recorded, as is the location of any pain that is produced.

With normal people the straight leg raise will usually be about 90°.

When I see patients with 'bad backs' I get them to 'straight leg raise' without my assistance. This is useful as they can note any losses and pain and monitor their own progress daily. *See Fig 31.*

The two techniques that I am about to describe, I use regularly on my patients with SLR restrictions. When they are helpful I teach the patients how to do them as part of their self treatment program. They are tried when there is no gross loss of 'straight leg raise' and pain with SLR is only in the buttock or above. What is more important is that when undertaken there must be no pain, and the outcome is an increase with SLR.

On the day of the patient's first visit, each technique is **only tried three times**. After that up to ten repetitions can be used.

If you are not happy with the following instructions or have any doubts about whether you should be using these techniques please seek the advice of a professional.

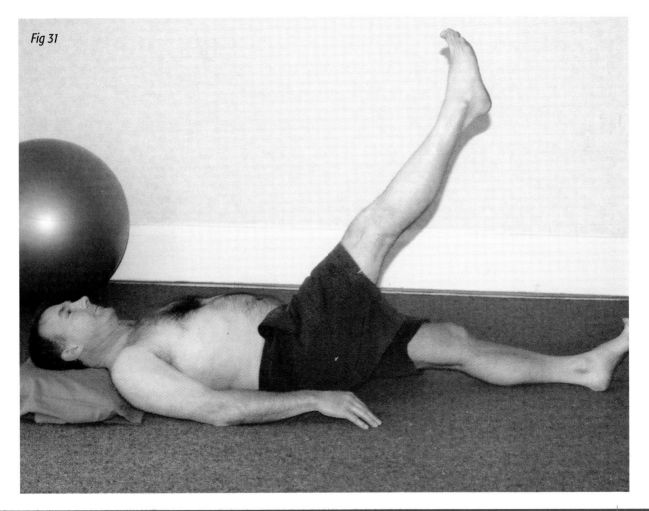

Fig 31

1. **The two leg rotation technique**. You lie on your back and grasp the side of the bed with your left hand if right 'straight leg raise' is limited. Both knees are now drawn up to chest. Your hips are carefully rotated to the right, which takes the bent up knees down to bed. Knees must remain flexed and no pain experienced. *See Fig 32* .

If there is discomfort this can often be eliminated by increasing or decreasing the amount of hip flexion. The hips are rotated in this way three times.

Remember no pain.

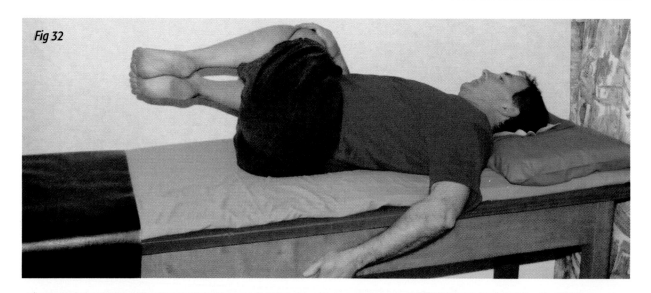

Fig 32

After these three rotations you retest your SLR. If the outcome is favourable then this technique can become part of your self-treatment routine on subsequent days. You can repeat the two leg rotations six times, several times a day if necessary.

Sometimes because of contact with your bed, you feel that you are not getting enough rotation. This can be increased by laying on top of two pillows. *See Fig 33.* These would lift the trunk above surface of the bed and allow more rotation.

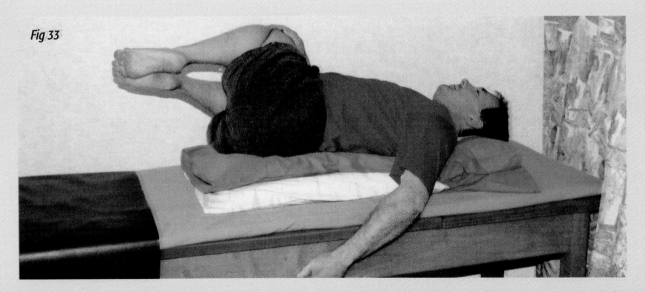

Fig 33

2. **The bent leg raise technique**. Lie on your back on the bed. Draw up knee to trunk on the side of the SLR limitation. Grasp bent leg behind knee. Now pull knee up and out from the side as far as you can, provided there is no pain. *See Fig 34.* This is done three times on day one and 'straight leg raise' is retested. If successful, on subsequent days, repeat six times, several times a day if necessary.

Another of the many technique that are available to me is called straight leg raise with traction. I will mention this later in the text as it has been shown to be extremely effective when used on people claiming to have "tight hamstrings".

Fig 34

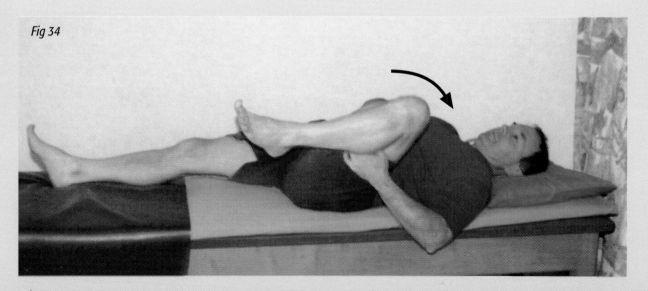

You will notice that I have put tight hamstrings in inverted commas. I do so as I believe that in many cases the inability to raise the straight leg fully is due to tightness in other structures and not due to a shortened hamstring. Anyway my technique has been shown to work more effectively than other published techniques in reducing "hamstring tightness". A reference for this can be found on my web-page.

When the techniques described above work in my clinic, I then ask the patient to do the two back exercises outlined below.

These two exercises are given to many of my patients with back pain even when their straight leg raise is normal.

I consider these exercises to be important as they take into consideration both components of each spinal segment. The passive back extensions deal with the disc component and the 'Lion' exercises deal with the facet joints.

The following exercises are in fact a copy of an exercise sheet that I give to my patients.

BACK EXERCISES

1. Passive back extensions (Half press ups):

Lie on your front with hands placed next to your chest. Keeping hips in contact with the ground, push your chest off the ground as far as possible (with no pain), then return to starting position. It is important that your arms do all the work, not the back muscles.

If pain is experienced, place hands closer to waist level and repeat.

For one-sided pain with this exercise place a pillow under your hip on the painful side. *See Fig 35.*

Stop if pain persists.

REPEAT 10X

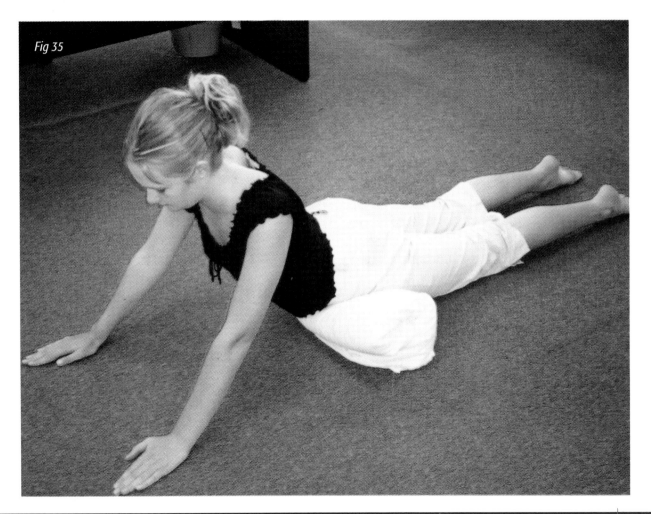

Fig 35

2. Lion exercises:

Kneel on all fours and place knees *wider apart* than shoulders. Keep arms straight and hands stationary, and move buttocks back towards your feet. Return to starting position.

REPEAT 10X

Alternatives:

• If painful, either hollow your lower back and repeat above, or hump lower back and repeat.

• If pain is more one sided, place knee on that side slightly closer to hands than the other. When moving backwards ensure you go straight back and not veer to side.

• For one-sided pain with this exercise place pad under knee on side of pain and then move buttocks towards your feet

Stop if not pain-free.

There is so much that can be done by way of treatment to the lumbar spine but that is not for inclusion in this book.

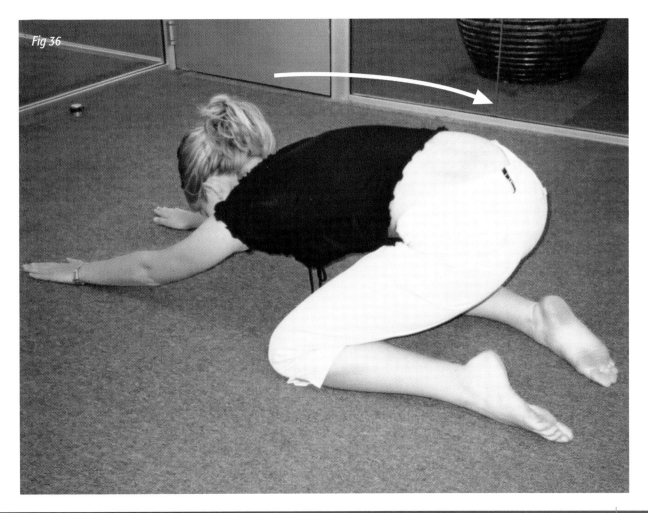

Fig 36

The Thoracic Spine

It is quite easy to strain your thoracic spine and such an event can cause considerable pain and movement restriction. You can upset this area in many ways. Awkward lifting, a fall, a violent sneeze or cough, a sudden rotation, jarring it when playing golf etc. etc. Pain can spread around chest wall from the level of involvement. When injured, and in the acute stage, pain will not only be increased with movement but with deep breathing as well. To cough or sneeze is so painful that patients soon learn not to do so and in fact as already mentioned a violent sneeze can injure your spine.

With chest pain, of course, the first thing that must be ruled out is heart pathology. Particularly if you experience left sided pain and the arm is involved.

Many conditions can give you thoracic pain. The gall bladder can cause pain between the shoulder blades and so on. Often chest pain without reason could result from shingles (herpes zoster) and not until the rash appears would this become obvious.

With chest pain it is wise to consult a medical practitioner to rule out serious pathologies.

Once it has been established that a strained thoracic spine is the cause of your symptoms you can try a self-traction to see if it makes you feel much better.

Before describing this, may I emphasize that the procedure must cause no discomfort at all. If it does, do not proceed.

Self-Traction for the Thoracic Spine.

You will require two chairs with standard height backs to them.

You have them facing away from each other with enough space between chair backs for you to stand between them. Now place a hand on the back of each chair. A small folded towel may be placed under each hand for comfort.

Keep your elbows straight and now bend your knees. Your toes will remain on the floor but your heels will lift off. As you sink down the tops of your shoulders will rise up in relation to your head. Most of the weight will be on the hands.

Relax your trunk and maintain the traction for 20 seconds. The spine should be vertical and not be extended.
See Fig 37.

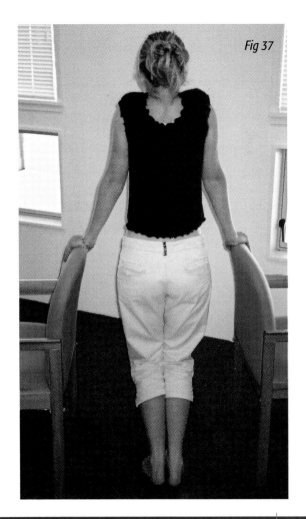

Fig 37

No pain should be felt. Repeat this stretch three times holding each one for 20 seconds.

After the third stretch you should be able to breath without discomfort if the technique is indicated.

After the third stretch you should be able to move more freely. You will not be 'cured' but feel easier.

This stretching can be repeated several times a day to speed up recovery or compliment any treatment that you are having on your spine.

I personally found that this form of traction enabled me to recover quickly from a low back strain I sustained lifting. This was because I applied a self-traction within minutes of straining my back.

The Sacro-Iliac Joints

These joints link the spine to the pelvis on each side. Their significance with regard to low back and hip pain is often ignored. Many patients are misdiagnosed as having a spinal problem causing their low back symptoms when in fact the culprit is the sacro-iliac joint (S/I joint). The treatment they are having is inappropriate and of course unsuccessful in dealing with their pain.

Within my concept there are many S/I mobilisations with movement techniques that practitioners can use on their patients. These techniques are useful in eliciting that the problem is with the sacro-iliac joint as well as treating it. In this publication I will explain one self-treatment that may be useful together with two other things that could be very helpful. However it would be better if you could see a practitioner who was familiar with my approach.

When your sacro-iliac joint is responsible for causing pain with bending backwards or leaning sideways to the painful side try repositioning your joint using a taping (sticking plaster) that is descibed below. While repositioning repeat the offending movements and see if the pain is absent. If there is NO PAIN you would then do 3 sets of 10, bending backwards and/or sideways.

After these repetitions you should find the offending movements are pain free. Repeat the exercises 6 times a day until you are better.

The self-treatment.

From your chemist buy a roll of firm 'Zinc Oxide' tape. It must be approximately 5 centimetres wide. See instructions to prevent skin reactions. *Page 88.*

Cut off a strip about 50 centimetres long. Attach half of this strip to the skin from the mid line so it lies across the upper buttock and wraps half way around your side. *See Fig 38*

Now fold the unattached end of the tape in half lengthways with the sticky side in to give you something to pull on. You grasp the free end of the tape with your hand on that side. Now pull forward strongly on the tape and arch backward (or sideways). Do not twist your trunk when pulling on the tape. If the movement is now pain free this is your self-treatment. Do the repetitions detailed above.

Many patients that I see with a sacro-iliac problem often have a slightly shorter leg on one side. If they do I have them place a piece of carpet in the heel of the shoe on that side to see if this helps.

When sitting aggravates a sacro-iliac lesion fold a small guest towel and place it under your buttock on the good side. This can often work wonders. It is well worth a try.

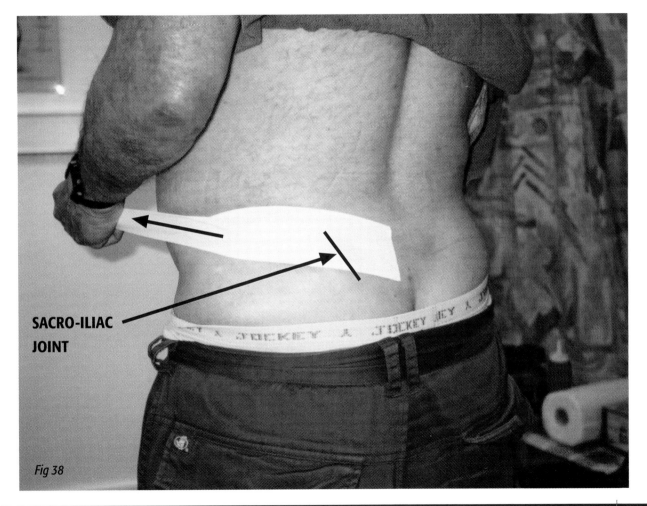

SACRO-ILIAC JOINT

Fig 38

Fingers

Everyone at some time seems to strain a finger. You could, miss-catching a basket ball for instance. Even when it is not fractured or visibly dislocated, but swollen and very stiff, it can be a proper nuisance. It can take a long time to settle.

Quite often when you reposition the joint surfaces, as to be described, you find that there is no pain and you can gain almost immediately the lost movement without discomfort. It really can be spectacular and traditional therapeutic procedures never bring about such a rapid recovery. I know because I have practiced for a long time this new approach of sustaining a mobilisation of the effected joint and combining it with movement ("MWM") and seen the minimal effects of other procedures that are regularly used.

A joint is where bones meet and movement take place. When you consider a finger joint, or **any** joint for that matter, the bone ends that meet are called facets. A proximal facet and a distal one. The proximal, by definition, is closer to the rest of the body when limbs are outstretched. With a finger the proximal facet is closest to palm.

Look at picture. *See Fig 39*

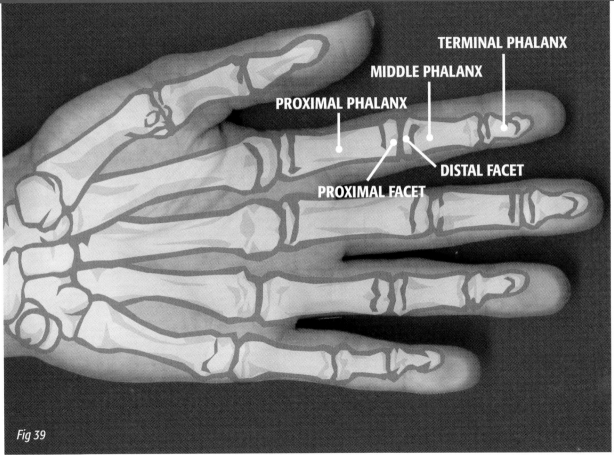

Fig 39

TERMINAL PHALANX

MIDDLE PHALANX

PROXIMAL PHALANX

DISTAL FACET

PROXIMAL FACET

I will explain what I do and perhaps you could get your partner to try this if you have a finger problem. If not get a therapist who knows of my approach to treat you.

When I see a patient with a painful swollen finger joint I place my thumb and index finger of one hand each side of the proximal facet of that joint and my other thumb and index finger each side of the distal facet. *See figure 40.*

I now, very gently, try to glide the distal facet sideways on the proximal facet.

It does not matter to which side you go because you will first try one way and then the other. With 90% of finger sprains you will find one direction painful and the other pain free. (I take care to glide the surface and not tilt it.)

The painful direction is taboo. I select and gently hold the facet in the pain free direction and then ask the patient to bend the sore finger joint while I maintain the glide. Movement should now be possible and without discomfort if the treatment is indicated. I then get patient to repeatedly flex and extend, while I maintain the corrective glide, ten times (remember no pain). After ten repetitions finger movement should be much better.

The thing to remember is that as the finger bends you must move your thumb and index finger with the moving section to sustain accurately the glide (repositioning).

To enhance the procedure I always get the patient, when she/he has bent the finger as far as possible, to passively push movement further with his/her free hand if it does not hurt.

It is so satisfying, with such a simple technique, to be able to instantly achieve so much.

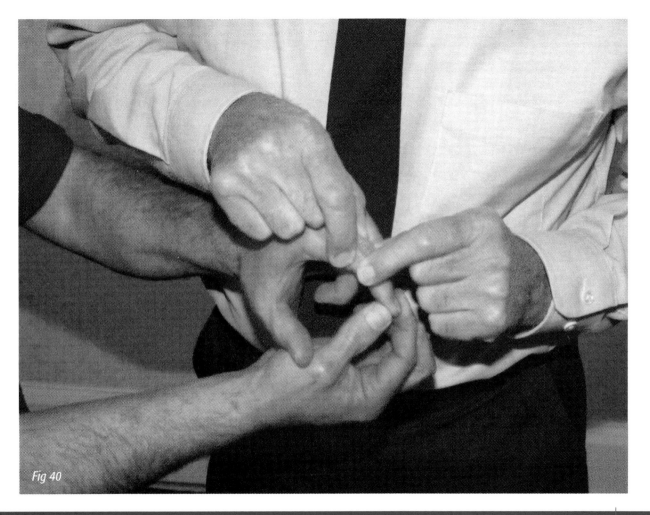

Fig 40

You will note, that I mentioned above, that 90% of finger strains have this interesting phenomenon where one side gliding direction is pain free and the other painful.

If both directions are painful then fix the proximal facet as you did before with one thumb and index finger. Now take the distal facet and turn (rotate) it in one direction and then the other. If one way hurts and the other doesn't then choose pain free rotation and ask patient to bend the finger.

Maintain the rotation while the finger bends and straightens. Repeat ten times with patient giving overpressure. By overpressure, I mean that the patient uses his free hand to bend finger further than he can actively bend it.

If above procedures cause pain irrespective of the repositioning of the joint surfaces do not proceed. See your health professional.

The whole philosophy behind mobilisations with movement is so simple and gentle and if you follow the 'no pain at all' rule you cannot go wrong. Remember it is not the panacea for all restricted joints.

Toes, especially the big toe, will respond just like fingers.

The Thumb

Many people have problems with the base of their thumbs. The sketch will show the area of pain. *See Fig 41.*

The pain is experienced when using it and after use it will often ache for some time. Taping the base of the thumb can make a great difference. If it is useful, re-tape it every day for a week or so until it has settled down.

I use a narrow (2 centimetres) piece of zinc oxide tape. One end of this is attached to the base of the thumb as the picture shows and the other end is pulled across the palm and attached. *See Fig 42.* It twists the bone inwards at the base and when the technique is indicated the thumb will move without pain. If painful, tape it the other way and see if this works. If not this approach is not used.

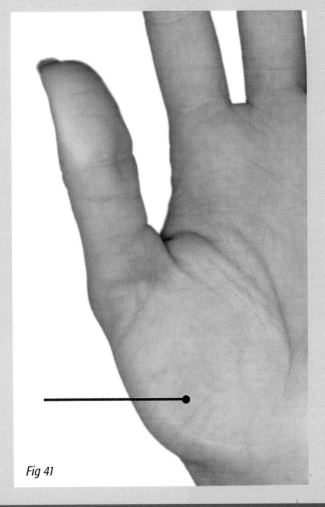

Fig 41

Another tip.

If the base of your thumb is aching grasp the thumb with your free hand and apply a very, very gentle traction for 20 seconds.
See Fig 43.

Provided the direction is right, you will often find the ache stops. When it does hold the traction for as long as you can and repeat a few times. The ache should stay away until you again do something to upset it.

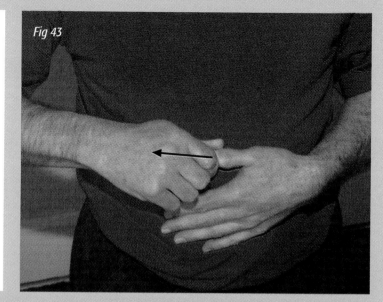

Fig 43

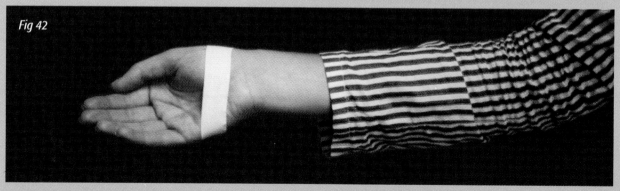

Fig 42

The Shoulder

I would like to begin by listing some things that you **should not** do with your shoulder.

Many people with normal shoulders can end up in misery with shoulder pain from a simple car activity. The shoulder joint is very vulnerable, when the elbow is at shoulder height and the hand is taken backwards and/or rotated.

It is the sort of thing that we often do when trying to pick something off back seat of a car whilst sitting in the front seat. **Please never do this**. It can lead to tendon damage in the shoulder. When the tendon is strained in this way it can be extremely painful and sometimes it takes a long time to recover. It can often leave the joint weakened so that the problem can reoccur.

Every year we see patients who strain their shoulders in the gym, lifting weights attached to the ends of a bar. They have the weighted bar they are clenching, lie across their shoulders, behind the neck. No, no, no! In this position the elbows are almost at shoulder height and stretched backwards. Similar to the starting position just discussed above when reaching behind you in the car.

Added to this, the head is forced to jut forward to keep it out of the way. In this hazardous starting position they now try to raise the heavy bar. For some shoulders and necks this stress is too much and problems in shoulders and/or neck can result.

Please keep bar in front of your head to eliminate most of the risk.

Many people with stiff shoulders are encouraged to do exercises and this is great, provided they do not make things worse.

A common exercise to help free a shoulder joint is called the pendulum exercise. Firstly you flex your hips so that your trunk is parallel to the floor. Now you are told to swing your arm to and fro and around in a circle. OK, but never do this with a weight in your hand.

A weight pulls the head of your upper arm bone (humerus) forward in its socket and will usually make you worse. *See Fig 44.*

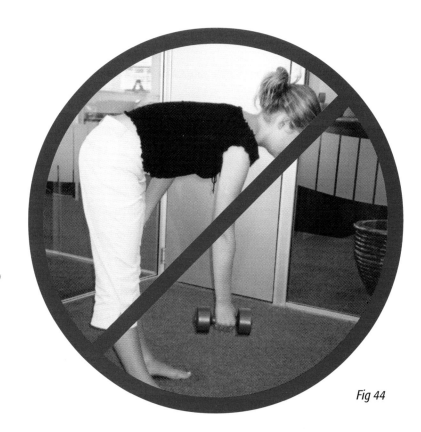

Fig 44

Most people with chronic shoulder problems are found to have the head of the humerus ever so slightly forward in the socket provided for it. The socket is part of the shoulder blade (scapula). To move it further forward by holding a weight in hand is silly and should be avoided.

If you want to increase a restricted range of movement forward and up, try the following.

Stand beside a table and place your hand on the restricted side flat on the table with your fingers pointing forwards. Keep your elbow straight and lean gently on your hand.

This slides the head of your humerus back in its socket. Keep the hand pressing on the table and step backwards, progressively bending at the hips as you do so. Go as far back as you can. *See Fig 45.*

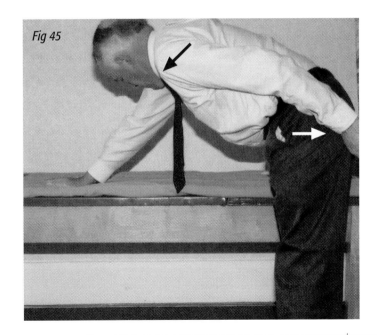

Fig 45

No pain should be felt and doing this should see a small increase in the range of movement. Repeat ten times and do these sets of 10 several times a day. If painful, stop!

Another way is to exercise the shoulder while lying on your back. Gravity helps to keep the bones in a better position. If you grasp a pole (broom stick) with both hands you can use your good arm to assist keeping the humerus in position while stretching above head. *See Fig 46*. Keep your shoulder blade from lifting off the bed.

OFTEN PAIN WITH ARM MOVEMENT CAN COME FROM A PROBLEM IN THE NECK

If you can, consult a therapist who is familiar with my techniques called 'Spinal mobilisations with arm movement' (SMWAM).

It can be an exciting approach and you can be taught to do this at home, when it proves to be successful. When indicated it brings about a rapid recovery and I know of no other techniques that can produce a quicker result. I just had to mention this. (Proof of its efficacy on patients is shown in a technical video that I produced but this is only available to the practitioners.)

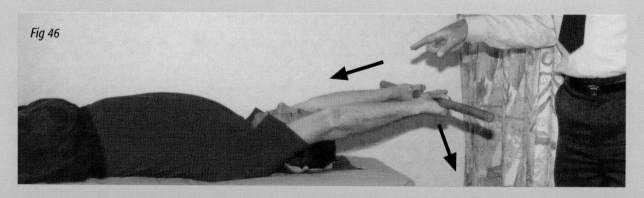

Fig 46

The basis of this approach is that when, for example, the fourth spinous process at the back of the neck is moved across to the left it opens the facet joint between fourth and fifth cervical (neck) vertebrae on right side. *See Fig 47.*

While this opening is being maintained the arm is then moved to see if pain with that movement is now eliminated. *See Fig 48.* When correct level is chosen and the arm is able to move without pain then the 'mobilisation with movement' is repeated six times. After these repetitions there should be a marked improvement in function.

Patients are taught to repeat this procedure several times a day and should be delighted with daily progress. *See Fig 49.*

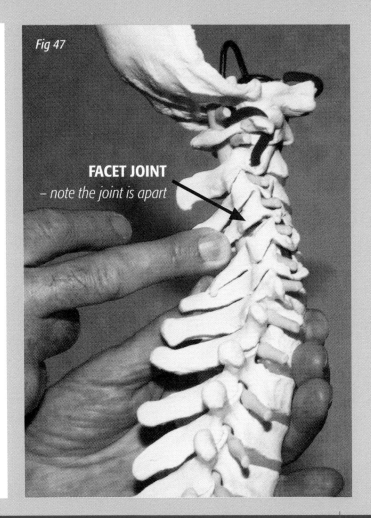

Fig 47

FACET JOINT
– note the joint is apart

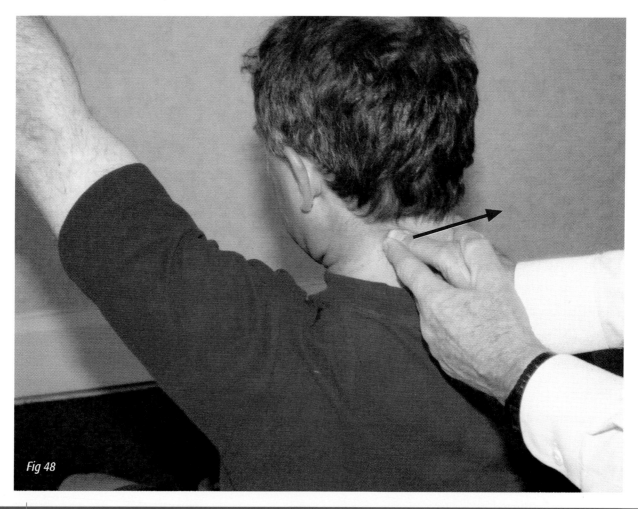

Fig 48

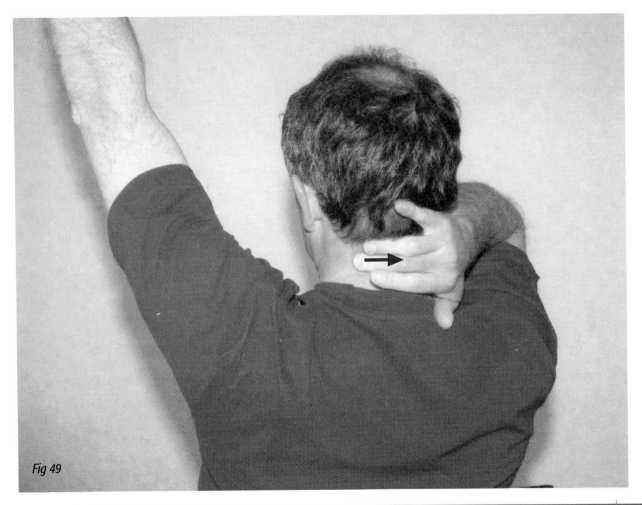

Fig 49

Heel Pain

Many people suffer from heel pain. It is sometimes called **plantar fasciitis**.

The heel pain that I am referring to is worse when you first arise in the morning or after sitting for a while and then getting up. It eases after walking for a while but if you walk too far it hurts again. . Apart from exercises and pertinent foot mobilisations, I have for many years used a special taping for heel pain. The results have been rewarding.

I will describe the taping and if you try it and it is successful you could go to a therapist, to have your sub-talar joints mobilised and ask them to give you appropriate sub-talar exercises. They will know, and explain, what is meant by the term sub-talar.

To tape the foot you will need 'Zinc Oxide' tape that is about 2 cms wide ($^1/_2$ inch).

See instructions to prevent skin reactions. *Page 88.*

You sit and place the foot with heel pain on your knee. You now wrap one end of tape under the heel. You now raise your heel up with one hand so that some creases in the skin appear between the heel and the inner ankle bone. Now wrap the tape obliquely across the ankle and up and around the lower leg. *See Fig 50.* You will need to use a second piece of tape over the top to strengthen it.

It is meant to feel strange when you first try to walk with the tape on. However after a few minutes of walking the tape will stretch a little and feel fine.

Leave it on and when you get up the next morning you should feel no pain. If it makes no difference then the taping is not for you. Keep looking for some other solution.

Daily taping and exercises may be needed for up to three weeks.

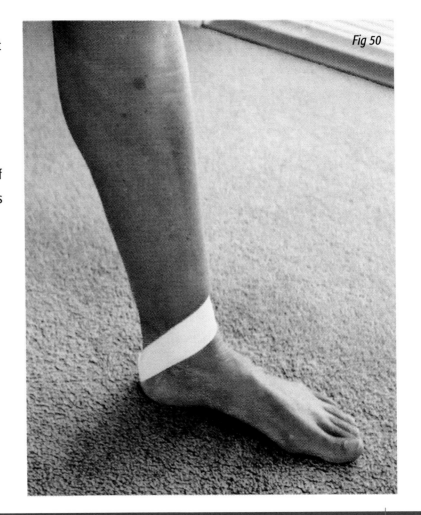

Fig 50

The Sprained Ankle

The ankle sprain is the commonest sporting injury in New Zealand.

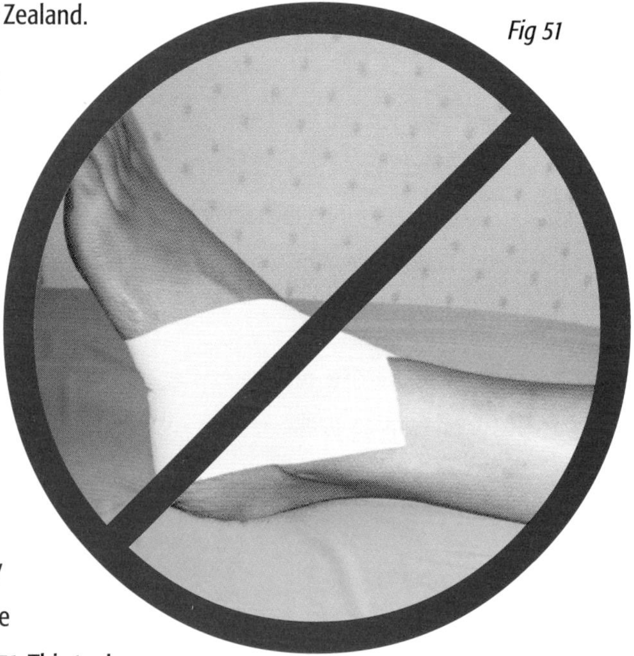

This occurs when the foot gets twisted violently down and inwards. You roll over on the ankle.

One sport that plays havoc with the ankle is netball. I guess that this is because when a player, who may be running at speed, receives the ball she is only allowed to take one step before passing it on. This sudden deceleration results in many ankles giving way.

The acute 48hour management of the injury using ice, compression, rest and elevation is fine. (R.I.C.E.)

However most of the tapings that are applied are generally dreadful. The foot is usually strapped in such a way that the 'victim' cannot turn his/her foot in, or flex it away. *See Fig 51.* This taping should rarely, if ever, be used. Restricting the normal movement and walking pattern with tape in this manner slows down the recovery and does not address what is usually the main problem, the ankle joint itself.

Fig 51

I believe that most of the damage with an inversion sprain occurs because the end of the fibula (the bone on the outside of the ankle) is wrenched forward on the tibia. This causes some chaos in the joint between lower end of tibia and fibula.

Now if the bottom end of the fibula is taped back on tibia the ankle joint feels spectacularly better.

I have found that the recovery time using this approach is halved and long-term outcomes are better.

It will be hard to explain the correct taping to the lay-person in a book like this and if you ever seek professional advice make sure that this person is aware of this new approach. Literature is starting to appear in different parts of the world supporting my hypothesis.

I considered myself an experienced teacher but became aware of my failings in a shattering way in 1998 when running a course in the USA. This course was a follow up course and all the participants had done courses with me before. When I got around to the ankle joint I asked the class if they were taping ankles my way and using my approach for ankle sprains. Only 6 out of 66 were. The others had had no success at all and had given the approach away. It turned out that my teaching was ineffective. It was a learning experience for me. I had taken too much for granted and not monitored accurately the performance of participants on courses to ensure that all had the techniques and taping right. They sure do these days.

My wife considered the paragraph above as unnecessary because it does not teach the reader anything. I begged to differ as getting the taping right is absolutely critical.

In this text I will explain the mobilisation with movements we do, but the emphasis will be on the correct taping.

If you have a sprained ankle problem and 24-48 hours has elapsed take this book to a therapist and seek advice or better still see someone who has done a course with me or with one of my accredited teachers.

TREATMENT APPROACH

When we see a patient who has sprained an ankle we lie her/him down and push the lower end of the fibula backward and up on the tibia. While we hold it in this position we ask her/him to turn the foot in. When done correctly there should now be no pain with this movement, whereas when this is attempted without this positional correction it is impossible because of pain.

To do this we place the padded part of our hand at the base of the thumb (the thenar eminence) on the lower end of the fibula and wrap our fingers around the back of the lower leg. *See Fig 52.* Our free hand lies under the lower end of the leg to support it. We push the fibula down and up (obliquely) on the tibia.

A piece of plastic foam over the end of fibula makes pressure on it more acceptable. This is important as initially the tissues are very very tender to touch.

We now have patient turn her/his foot down and in to see if she/he can now do so without pain. If it is painful keep slightly adjusting the direction of your force until the foot moves in, without pain. When pain free movement is achieved have patient repeat movement ten times while bones are held in this way. Three sets of this exercise are done.

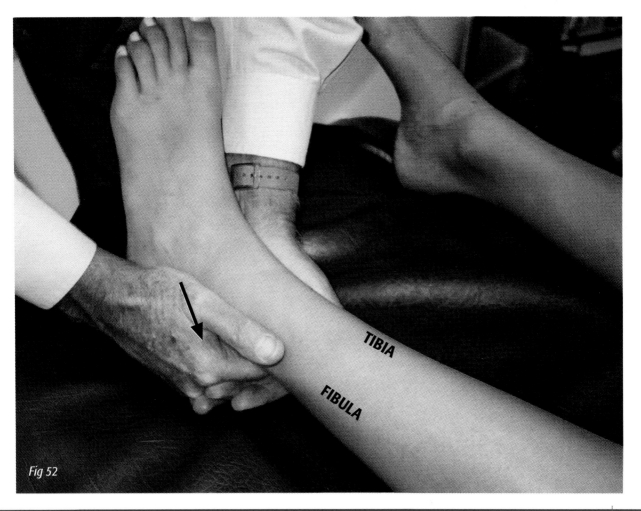

Fig 52

TIBIA

FIBULA

Remember the movement should produce no pain. There should be **no pain**. After this, the fibula is taped in the following way.

TAPING

Before applying any tape we ask if the patient is allergic to tape.

If he/she is not then the area to be taped is prepared by:

1. Shaving it. (Removing tape from a hairy surface is extremely painful and should be avoided.)

2. Using extra strength "Mylanta" antacid (this is really a stomach medicine taken to relieve indigestion) or a similar antacid product. The skin is 'painted' with it and left to dry. When it does, it leaves a white powder on the skin, which is rubbed off. The antacid on the skin neutralises the zinc oxide tape which is acidic and reduces the chances a skin reaction. I learned of this 'anointing' in the States a couple of years ago and what a wonderful assistance it has been.

If they are allergic to tape:

1. Try the "Mylanta" and remember to shave first.

2. Use one of those under-wraps that are currently on the market and stop the tape from making contact with the skin.

3. Try painting the skin with Friar's Balsam before taping. Keep this from clothing as it can stain it. N.B.Some people can be allergic to Friars Balsam. Do a small skin test first.

Although I can tape patients on my own it is better to have someone to assist.

You place tape as shown in sketch so that it lies obliquely over lower end of fibula leaving tip of this bone free. You now push back and up on the lower end of the fibula as explained earlier.

While repositioning in this way have a helper wrap tape firmly around lower leg as shown in picture. *See Fig 53.* They pull it down firmly and wrap it around obliquely.

Applying the tape to an ankle at the time of injury can be unpleasant because the tissues are so tender. However the patients will always forgive you as it enables them to walk much better.

If an injury has just occurred then you would first apply ice. After 20 minutes, tape and then wrap a pressure bandage over the top.

Never leave the tape on for longer than 48 hours. If, before this time has elapsed, they experience any skin irritation then it must be removed straight away.

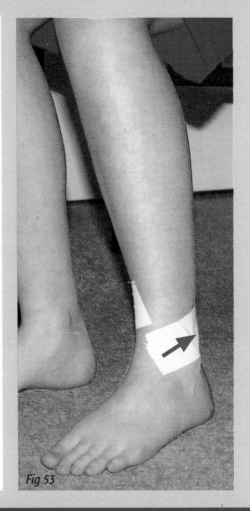

Fig 53

Removing the tape requires care. It is so easy to pull off a small piece of skin if you just 'rip it' off. After inspecting the skin, the ankle can be re-taped as you did before (another 48 hours).

Sometimes two days of taping is enough as the ankle feels much better but remember a joint has been injured so take things easy for at least fourteen days.

For those with weak unstable ankles, tape in the manner described before you play sport and remove it after the game.

You could try and tape your own ankle.

Place your foot with the sprained ankle on a chair. Now turn the foot in and knee out, which tends to place the lower end of the fibula back on the tibia, as we want it to be. The tape is now securely wrapped obliquely around the lower leg as detailed above. This way of taping was suggested to me by two therapists on a course of mine in Woolongong, Australia. *See Fig 54.*

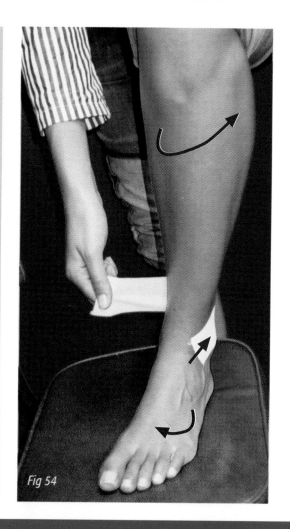

Fig 54

The Painful Knee

There are many reasons for knee pain and stiffness. Some are the result of injury, others due to wear and tear and others due to pathologies that need to be investigated.

However it may prove very beneficial to try the following test.

Place your foot on the sore knee side on the flat surface of a chair. With the knee of the other leg straight, lean forward over chair, which will bend sore knee further. You are doing this to see if it is painful and/or restricted.

If there is pain and a loss of movement try the following:

Let us assume that your right knee is the painful one.

Place your foot on the sore knee side on the flat surface of a chair.

Place the padded part at the base of your right thumb at the outer back the lower leg just below the right knee as shown in illustration. *See Fig 55.* Your right thumb lies beside the fingers, which are wrapped around the leg. Your left hand wraps around front of the lower leg just below right hand.

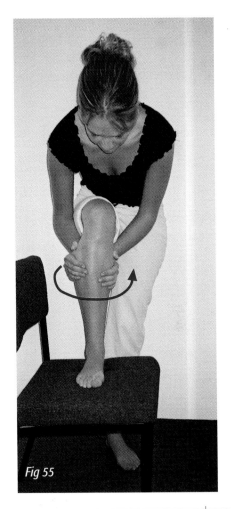

Fig 55

Now twist upper end of lower leg inwards on the knee. The foot is not turned in but stationary.

While maintaining this rotation, come forward over affected knee provided there is no pain and knee bends more freely.

This is one of the most useful tests that you can do for a knee. I say this, as if the pain goes and the knee bends much further the test now becomes a self-treatment.

As a treatment do up to three sets of 10 knee flexions with foot on chair. After three sets your knee should now be feel much better. Patients are told to repeat this self-mobilisation with movement at least four times a day. After a few days they should be much better. The success of this form of therapy is dependant on the routine described causing no discomfort at the time of delivery.

To speed up recovery the knee can be taped so that upper end of the lower leg (tibia and fibula) remains turned in on the thigh.

The taping to be described is also wonderful for patients who have pain under the kneecap with activities like running ('runners knee'), squatting down or climbing and descending stairs or sloping surfaces. (In the young it is called 'chondromalacia'.)

With these patients appropriate exercises should be done to strengthen inner part of thigh muscle.

However you should consult your medical advisor or therapist about these.

KNEE TAPING *(See comments about wiping skin over with MYLANTA etc. on page 88)*

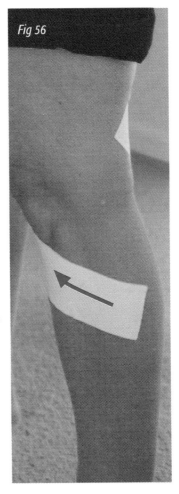

Fig 56

You will need to purchase 5 centimetre wide zinc oxide tape from the chemist.

Stand with your knee bent about 5 degrees.

One end of tape is placed obliquely around upper end of the lower leg. It lies halfway across the surface behind the upper lower leg, as you can see from the illustration. *See fig 56.* Now turn your foot in, keeping big toe in contact with floor. At the same time thigh is twisted in opposite direction. While this position is sustained pull the tape firmly up and around finishing half way around the back of the thigh.

The upper edge of the tape lies about 2 centimetres below kneecap as it crosses.

This taping procedure is not too difficult and can be done without assistance, but it is always easier if there is someone to help.

When indicated, tape each morning and remove it at night to prevent skin intolerance.

It may be necessary to tape for up to three weeks.

The two tapings that I have used the most in recent years are the knee taping above and the taping for the sprained ankle.

Trochanteric Bursitis

The thigh-bone (femur) runs slightly up and out from the knee and then changes direction up and in for about 10 centimetres to form the hip joint. If you look at the illustration you will see where bend occurs. *See sketch fig 57.* The bump at the side that you can feel, a spread hand width down from the waist, is called the great trochanter. Over this trochanter is a bursa called the trochanteric bursa. A band of gristle runs down outer side of leg passing over this bursa.

As we swing our leg to and fro, the bursa's role is to facilitate a smooth passage, over the trochanter, of the band of gristle.

Every year I see patients who for a variety of reasons have a swollen, painful bursa. It may be from a fall or knock, or occur spontaneously for whatever reason. The pain is local to the trochanter, felt when standing up or sitting down, climbing stairs and sometimes even when walking. It can be sore in bed when you lie on it.

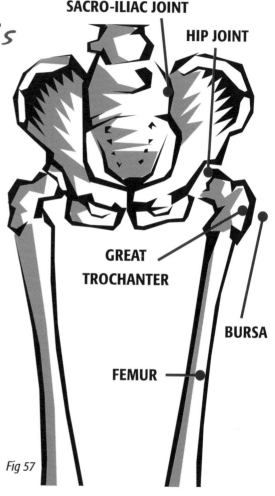

SACRO-ILIAC JOINT

HIP JOINT

GREAT TROCHANTER

BURSA

FEMUR

Fig 57

It usually responds well to therapy but there are two things that you can try if you have a problem.

Firstly use an ice pack for about 25 minutes. A medium size packet of frozen peas is ideal for this purpose. It can be applied twice a day. To protect the skin from an 'ice' burn rub some Vaseline on the area before applying the ice. If using crushed ice, put it in a damp towel so that the ice itself is not in direct contact with the skin.

The second suggestion is to tape the upper leg.

In addition to applying ice you can tape the area so that the effect of the band of gristle passing back and forth over the bursa with leg movement is altered.

If taping is going to be useful, you know as soon as it is applied. The movement pain goes or is markedly reduced. Because the bursa is not now being irritated with leg movement all the time, it settles quickly in a few days.

Remember that tape must not cause any irritation and must never be left on for longer the 48 hours. If it causes the area to itch or burn remove it straight away. Read my earlier comments about the use of tape on page 88.

You need tape that is 5 centimetres wide and long enough to reach from behind the buttock, just above the trochanter, to just past the middle of your abdomen.

You firstly attach one end of the tape half way across the buttock so tape's lower edge is about 3 centimetres above the trochanter.

Now pull tape forward and slightly upwards which takes muscle mass forward and then wrap it around your abdomen as shown in diagram. *See Fig 58.*

Ideally remove tape each night and re-tape each morning until bursa has settled.

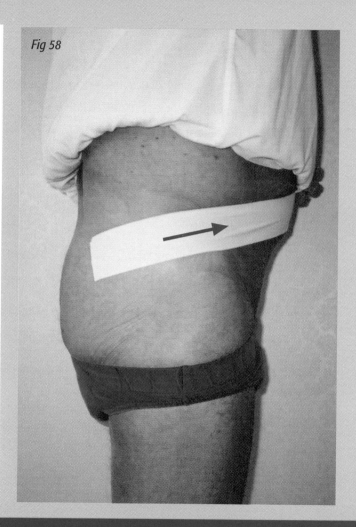

Fig 58

"Tight Hamstrings"

A published study from Curtin University in Perth, Australia, showed that the technique that I initially used for certain spinal problems appears to 'stretch the hamstrings' more effectively than other current techniques that have been studied and published.

I believe that sportspeople especially hurdlers would find it extremely useful.

Earlier in the section on the lumbar spine I said that apparent tightness in hamstrings is probably due to other structures.

Let me explain the technique then you, the reader, can draw your own conclusions.

Someone else does the stretching so it cannot be called a self-treatment but it must be included in this text because of its proven value.

The person with the "tight hamstring" lies on the floor.

If it is a left hamstring the person doing the stretch (stretcher) stands on the left and grasps leg at ankle. A comfortable way to do this is to have back of the lower leg, lie in the bend of the "stretcher's" elbow. Their other hand secures the leg in the elbow. Photo will show grip. *See Fig 59.*

Now the "stretcher" applies a longitudinal traction in the direction indicated by the arrow on the photo. *See Fig 60.*

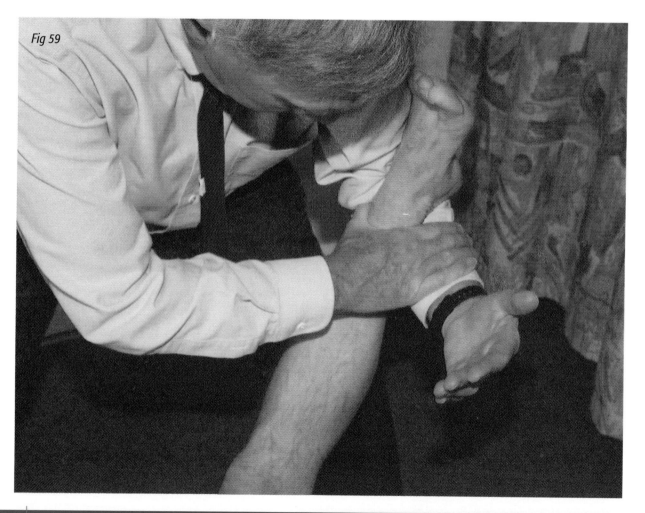

Fig 59

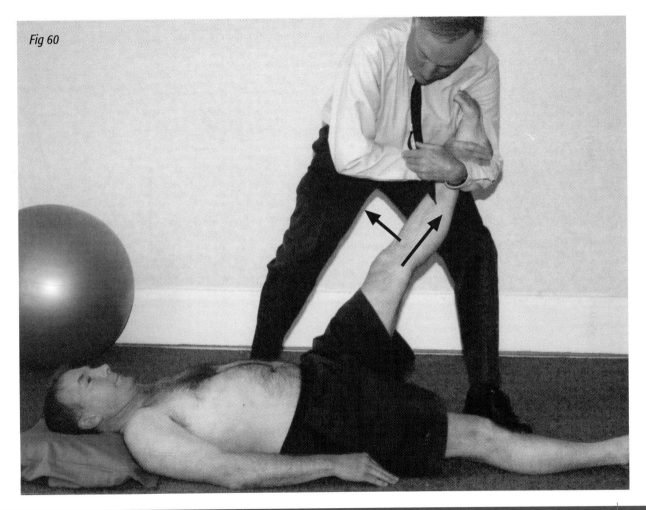

Fig 60

The leg is raised up and out from side as far as it will go with no pain. If it hurt you would abandon the technique. When being raised, the hip on that side would almost be off the floor.

Never let traction off until the leg is lowered to the starting position.

Three of these stretches should produce an immediate change in the straight leg raise range if the technique is going to be of value.

When it is, another seven stretches could be done.

If the stretch appears ineffective it could mean that you may not have applied sufficient traction or taken the leg out from the side when stretching.

The interesting observation that one finds is that when an un-stretched leg is raised to its limit a stretch is always felt in the hamstring. When the above technique is applied no tight feeling in the hamstring is felt until the leg is much higher.

This leads me to believe that the tightness is in other structures causing the hamstring to be unreasonably and prematurely stretched. The traction releases these other structures and thus the good result. (If my supposition is wrong, so what, the technique works and has been proved to do so.)

Just remember **NO PAIN**.

Muscle Strains

MWMS involve repositioning joint surfaces to see if this action enables pain free function to occur.

A similar approach can be used with muscle strains. We all know that when we strain a muscle we should ice it, apply a pressure bandage, rest it for 24 hours and keep it elevated to control swelling. Physical therapy is the treatment of choice.

Damaged muscle fibres can be positioned with tape to see if this reduces the pain that is initially felt when the muscle is contracted. If it does taping should be part of the treatment regime.

As an example let us consider the patient who has torn some muscle fibres in his calf muscle. When this sort of injury occurs it is usually fibres on the inner side of the muscle that are involved. Take a strip of 5 centimetre wide sports tape. (Remember the rules for taping) Now place one end of the strip across the calf muscle bulk at the level of the muscle damage.

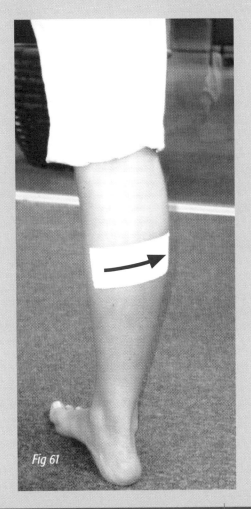

Fig 61

Hold the tape firmly and pull it out and the wrap it around the leg. *See Figure 61.*

This changes the shape and position of the muscle bulk so that the inner side of the calf muscle is slightly concave. This taping shortens the muscle where the strain has occurred and can make it feel much more comfortable with walking etc. If it does, tape it in this way in the morning, remove the tape at night and repeat the procedure for several days until the leg has healed. If it made no difference do not use the taping.

If the damage to the muscle is on the outer side of the calf then the tape should be applied pulling the muscle bulk inwards.

This repositioning of muscle bulk with tape can be tried for any muscle strain to see if it is helpful.

Pain Release Phenomenon Techniques [PRPS]

These are sometimes indicated for limbs.

It is with some trepidation that I write of these procedures because all advice and techniques in this publication up to this point stress that you should experience **no pain**.

I now want to share an interesting discovery that I made by sheer accident many years ago.

I was seeing a patient with a long-standing elbow problem. His symptoms were bizarre when compared with textbook conditions that beset the elbow and forearm. For 18 months he was unable to turn his right forearm clockwise, when any power was required, because of pain. He could not use a screwdriver for instance. He had other painful signs and symptoms that did not make sense.

As a final test I asked him to rotate his forearm clockwise while gripping my hand. I moderately resisted this movement while he did so and it provoked his pain. He sustained this motion against my resistance for some time while we were talking and made the observation after about 20 seconds that the pain he had been experiencing had gone.

Many years ago Louis Pasteur wrote, "In the field of discovery chance only favours a prepared mind". I guess that on that day my mind must have been prepared. I immediately asked the patient to relax for a moment and I again applied some resistance through my hand-grip to his forearm rotation.

The pain was again provoked at a tolerable level and to my astonishment after about 20 seconds it had gone. Then things started to change. Further resisted pain producing movements saw the time for the pain to stop, start dropping. It would go in 15 seconds then 10 then 5 and then to provoke any discomfort considerable resistance to his forearm rotation was required. Within minutes his rotation movement under load was pain free.

This then made me stretch his elbow in the direction that had been painful, provoke an acceptable level of discomfort and sustain it to see what would happen. "Magic"! Would you believe that within 20 seconds his pain had gone with the stretch. Repetitions saw the similar pain reduction behaviour that was encountered with the forearm rotations.

After some minutes the patient **was unable** to reproduce the pains that he came in with.

I sent him home with instructions to repeat the provocation of his elbow signs if he could. He was to sustain any painful activities at a tolerable level and see if they would go. If they did he was to repeat the routine that we went through.

When he returned two days later he was virtually symptom free. We were both delighted as he had had this problem for 18 months. A subsequent call confirmed he had made a complete recovery.

Interesting? It certainly was to me. This got me thinking about chronic soft tissue pain and whether we had stumbled upon yet another approach that could be applied with safety when conventional approaches had failed.

For nearly two decades I have used this approach of sustained tolerable pain provocation with great success on LONG STANDING painful wrists, shoulders, hips, thumbs, knees and so on. The danger of writing about it is that if care is not taken to follow the rules necessary with this form of treatment a condition can be made worse for a few days.

So to start with I would like to give you some rules for the application of "PRPS" and examples of their use to assist you to understand more about them.

RULES

1. Do not try PRPS on acute conditions. They will not work.

   They are for conditions of longer than 6 weeks duration.

   They will probably be useless if the problem has been present for over two years but are still worth a try.

2. The treatment as the name suggests, involves first of all provoking the pain that you, the patient, is being troubled by.

   The pain may be provoked by joint movement, compression of a joint with movement, or a muscle contraction.

   (An example of compression of a joint with movement would be pressing down on a knee cap and then gliding ('grinding') the knee cap over the bones beneath.) This pain must be MILD and NEVER STRONG. If provoked strongly the condition can be made worse.

3. Sustain the stretch or compression with movement or resistance that produces this mild level of pain and check with a watch to see if the pain disappears within 20 seconds. If it does not then you would not use the technique.

   However check that you have not provoked too much pain initially. That may be the reason why the pain did not go in 20 seconds. To be sure, provoke a lesser pain and wait 20 seconds just in case. If the pain goes within say 5 seconds you have probably been too gentle, so repeat the procedure using a stronger provocation. Remember that when successful, after four or five repetitions the time for the pain to stop will start dropping and the 'force' required to produce it will need to be increased. After a few minutes the condition should feel "heaps better".

   You can treat yourself daily if you are able to manage the self-pain provocation.

   Ideally, the treatment should be initiated by a therapist familiar with "PRPS" or you will need to show them the details in this book. Please adhere strictly to the 20 second rule.

4. "PRPS" are not for children or the frail and old.

5. Do not use them on people with whom you cannot converse. (They may speak another language.) The patient must be fully aware of what you are about to do and have the intelligence to cooperate.

EXAMPLES OF HOW "PRPS" MAY BE APPLIED

1. Pain under the kneecap (patella)

If you are under 50 years and have been bothered for some time with pain under the kneecap, which has not responded to medication, therapy, taping etc. then a "PRP" may be useful. Sit up on a couch or bed with a pillow under your knee. Place the palm of one hand over kneecap and place other hand on top. Now push down on your kneecap to compress the surfaces underneath. *See Fig 62.* This should not cause pain. Now while sustaining the compression move the kneecap to and fro in different directions seeking out a painful response. If a particular motion is painful keep moving back and forth in this manner provoking the pain at a TOLERABLE level.

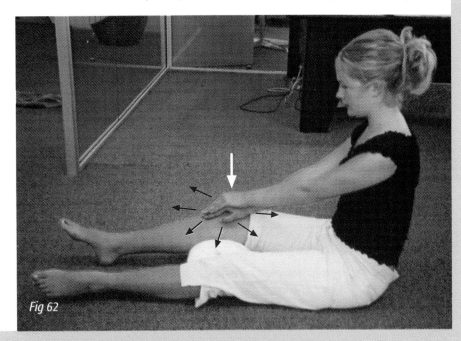

Fig 62

Within 20 seconds of starting this repetitive motion with compression the pain should have gone. If not then you may have provoked too much pain. Try again with less compression. If still sore stop because this technique is not appropriate.

If the pain does go in 20 seconds, rest for about 5 seconds and repeat the "PRPS". Again the pain must go with in 20 seconds. After several repetitions the pain will go off sooner and within minutes there should be no pain at all with the treatment.

You may need to go through this routine for several days until the knee is feeling normal again.

Remember if on the first try the pain goes in say 8 seconds apply a bit more compression force.

Another point with the knee is that several different directions may be painful. If so, clear one and then move on to another and so on.

2. Hip pain

When there is a problem with the hip joint there is a test that is done which when positive confirms that the hip is not normal. It is called "Fabers test". You lie on back, bend up knee on sore side and place outer side of your ankle just above opposite knee. Leaving ankle where it is take knee on sore side down to the bed. If movement is restricted and painful with overpressure down when using your hand on that side to push it down, you have a hip joint problem. *See Fig 63.*

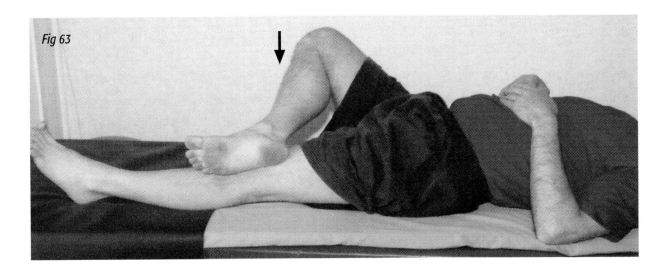

Fig 63

You can compare the range of movement with the other side. If your hip pain is chronic then try a "PRP". Sustain the pressure down with your hand and see if the pain goes in 20 seconds. Remember not to cause too much pain. If the pain goes, then go through "PRP" treatment routine.

3. Shoulder pain

 When you have a problem with your shoulder the pain always radiates down the arm, which can be misleading. If you have not responded to conventional treatment a "PRP" may be the answer. (They have no place if your shoulder has stiffened. This restricted shoulder is often called a 'frozen shoulder' and "PRPS" are useless.)

Try this.

Lie on your back, bend elbow and take it in the direction of the opposite shoulder. Now place the palm of your free hand over your elbow and push obliquely down. *See Fig 64* The direction is along the shaft of your upper arm bone. (Humerus) . Keep altering the direction slightly and see if you can provoke shoulder pain. If you can, sustain the pressure down on the elbow to see if the pain goes off in the magical 20 seconds. If it does you are "in business".

Often with these techniques you can get your partner to do the work, however as the procedure is complicated you should ideally get a professional to do this.

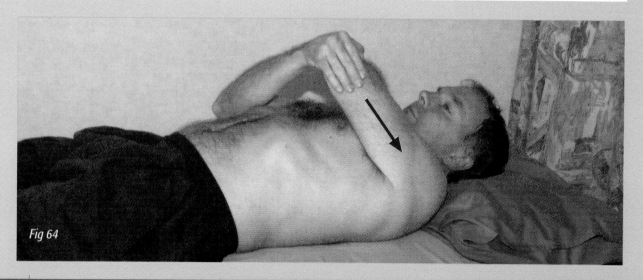

Fig 64

4. Chronic wrist pain

Sometimes with overuse, the wrist can cause a great deal of trouble and it is difficult to fix. Computer use is one cause of wrist pain.

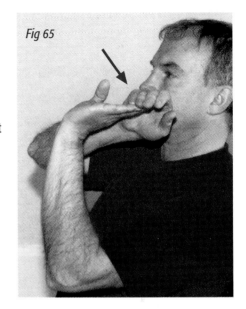

Fig 65

Let us assume that you have had longstanding wrist pain. The pain is felt when you flex or extend wrist and apply some overpressure.

"PRPS" should be tried and as any pain provocation must always be tolerable it will ensure the condition will not be made worse if it turns out that "PRPS" are of no value.

Bend your wrist backward and push with your other hand until it hurts. *See Fig 65.* Back off a little so that the hurt is acceptable and sustain the stretch for up to 20 seconds to see what will happen.

If the pain goes, you know that the treatment is indicated and will be of value. Do your repetitions in the manner already described until there is virtually no pain when you bend the wrist back.

Now bend it the other way and "PRP" it until that is also better.

I treated a woman recently with a 2 year history of wrist pain that had not responded to the many forms of treatment given by others including surgery. After three visits to me she was fine. In between her visits she did her own "PRPS".

5. De Quervains Disease

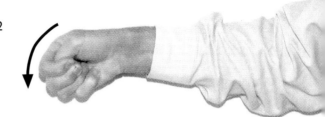

Fig 66

Another patient had what was called De Quervains disease for 2 years. She had had therapy, injections and finally surgery. She was no better, but after three visits with me her grip had returned, she was virtually pain free and able to return to work.

The lady in question had what was called a positive 'Finkelstein's test'. Because of sharp pain she was unable to bend her wrist sideways towards her little finger when she wrapped her fingers around her thumb. *See Fig 66.*

Fig 67

The "PRP" for her was in fact to provoke a small pain with the 'Finkelstein's test' and wait 20 seconds to see if it would go.

To make it work after such a long time we had to start with the wrist slightly bent forward. *See Fig 67.*

She was taught to treat herself between visits.

You will find that these treatments are not a panacea for all chronic soft tissue pain but should be considered as an option when all else has failed. Remember they are moderate enough to do no harm when they fail.

6. Base of thumb

Many of us get some wear and tear (osteoarthritis) in the joint at the base of the thumb. This can be a real nuisance when we have to grip things to lift them or even gripping a pen for instance. Try a "PRP" procedure.

A useful approach is to grab the thumb with your other hand and push down along the shaft to compress the joint at the base of the thumb. Now, while sustaining the compression, passively flex and extend thumb (across palm and back) and see if this is painful. *See Fig 68.* If it is, move the thumb back and forth under acceptable compression and see if pain goes in, yes, 20 seconds. If it does, carry on with repetitions.

When flexion and extension is OK try bending the thumb away from the palm and back under compression and see if that is sore. If it is treat it. Quite often both directions are sore anyway so you would treat in both directions.

I could go on and on but I consider that I have given sufficient examples for the use of "PRPS" that should enable you, the reader, to experiment a little. But please follow the rules and be sensible.

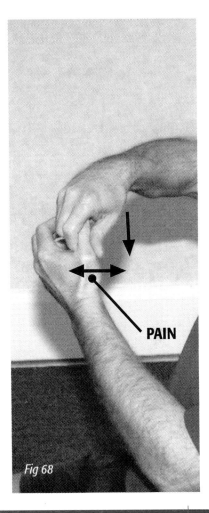

PAIN

Fig 68

THIS LITTLE BOOK SHOULD PROVE HELPFUL

When you have ongoing musculo-skeletal problems remember there is a lot of help 'out there'. It is a matter of knowing where to look.

When we have chronic pain that is not responding to orthodox medicine we seek help from those practitioners on the fringe. Some are opportunists preying on the vulnerable, but, casting those aside, there are many people who are practising successfully because they have something to offer.

Manual therapy for instance is the treatment of structures by mechanical means such as mobilisation or manipulation to relieve pain and restore function.

If you are being treated with mobilisation or manipulation you should always leave the premises of the practitioner feeling better than when you arrived. This of course is a generalisation but a pretty good guide.

I have had patients tell me that they have been to people who have told them they have put "things back" and that they will now settle slowly. The patient is often in agony but believes the old adage it has got to get worse before it gets better. When it settles some time later they believe that this was because of their treatment. Very unlikely.

The chances are that it recovered anyway. Actually it may have taken a little longer because of inappropriate manhandling.

Remember after treatment you should leave feeling better than you were beforehand.

Always ask for a good explanation from the person treating you as to what they believe is your problem and how they propose to help. Do not let them baffle you.

Also request a treatment time frame. Beware of the practitioner who over treats.

And remember the average bad back for instance, is usually better anyway within six weeks, if not sooner.

Many, once you are in their clutches, will suggest frequent follow up treatments to ensure your 'well-being'. The more you manipulate a joint the more unstable it may become. I have used manipulation for over thirty years and it is an excellent treatment tool. However by definition you manipulate a joint when you force it to move beyond its normal physiological range. It is not a natural movement so should not be done too often.

Finally, the self-treatment advice that I have given must bring about a change at time of delivery. If not discard it just like you should discard any practitioner who is not bringing about some immediate improvement when using manual therapy for mechanical pain.

INDEX

NOTES